Contents

Introduction: 4
A Brief History: 6
My Journey 11
The Bottom Line - Kill the Cancer Stem Cells 13
PubMed® 15
Bharat B. Aggarwal, PhD 18
Doctor Bradford Weeks M.D. 20
Max Wicha 25
It Make Sense: Anti-Inflammatory and Cancer Stem Cells 27
$$$The Bottom Line $$$ 29
What Happens If You Don't' Kill the Cancer Stem Cells 30
Reactive vs Proactive 32
Falling into the Trap: Pharmaceutical vs Natural Products 34
Are There Other Ways to Kill Cancer Stem Cells? 35
    The Keto Diet 35
    Cannabis Oil/CBD 36
    Melatonin 36
    Targeting Cancer Stem Cells by Melatonin 37
    High Dosages Melatonin 38
    IP-6 39
    Metformin 40
Inflammation to be Avoided 41
Glucose 45
How I Killed the Cancer Stem Cells 48

Generally Recognized as Safe (GRAS) 50
Understanding FDA Food Labels 53
Recipes 57
The Gift That Will not Stop Giving: Chemotherapy and Radiation 60
Apoptosis 61
My Treatment Plan 61
There Is No Cure For Cancer 64
Glioblastoma Multiforme 65
Ludwig Center 68
Backup 69
    Garlic 69
    Turmeric/Curcumin 70
    Ginger 73
    Cayenne Pepper 75
    Black Seed Oil 76
    Cinnamon 82
    Avocado 85
    Blueberries 86
    Strawberries 88
    Coconut Oil 89
    Olive Oil 90
    Oatmeal 91
    Coffee 91
    Red Meat 93
    Bread 95
    Gluten 97
    Keto Diet 98
    Cannabis Oil/CBD 100
    Melatonin 106

High Dose Melatonin	114
IP-6	125
Photos	130
Cancer Parks	135
Stem Cells vs Cancer Stem Cells From Wikipedia	139
Wikipedia Defines Cancer Stem Cells	140
My MRI's:	143

Introduction:

Cancer is a chronic metabolic disease. Chronic diseases can be controlled, not cured. There is no cure for cancer. We all have cancer cells in our bodies.

This is dedicated to my Mom, Helen JoAnn McCraw. She died of Pancreatic Cancer on 10/08/2012

Disclaimer: I am not a Doctor. I am a survivor of a Glioblastoma Multiforme Grade 4 Brain Tumor. For those that don't know it is a Brain Tumor. I have done a lot of research. This is my story, and I am sticking to it. This is what I believe. I believe that the key to beating cancer lies in the *__Cancer Stem Cells__*.

For the latest information go to my website:*beatingthecancer.com*

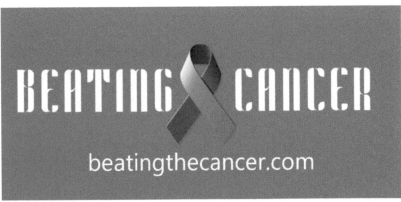

Email: james_mccraw@beatingthecancer.com

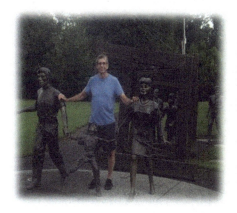 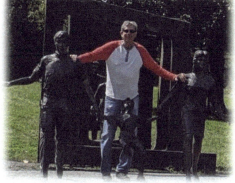

          April 11, 2018   *June 1, 2020*

A Brief History:

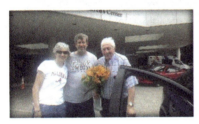

Figure 1 *my sister, me, my dad*

I was living in Dallas, Tx when I got the tumor and had all my treatments at Dallas Baylor. In November 2013 I had to move back to Memphis, Tn where I could be closer to family. I could not drive because a seizure. I could not work because of the cancer. It was not until December 2013 before I could do research on GBM. After the surgery, on October 13, 2013, I was a mess. I had trouble with loud sounds. I had trouble logging in to the internet. I was unable to talk more than a few words. (If you don't count the cusswords) my vocabulary was extremely limited. I could not put words or thoughts together. I was a blank slate. I had trouble telling time. Common words I could not say. It still happens today but it is better. If I say them over and over until I could eventually say them. Right now, I can't say Brussel Sprouts.

I had an awake craniotomy; the Surgeon thinks he got half of the tumor, but it was too bloody to tell. Chemotherapy, called Temozolomide (it's also known as Temodar), and Radiation simultaneously. My last day of Radiation was October 29, 2013. The last of day Temodar Phase 1 - 150 mg was October 23, 2013. I finished the Temodar 2nd Round from January 1, 2014, until May 5, 2014. In round #2 they bumped up the dosage to 3 x (140) MG. You had to take it for the first five days for 5 months. May 5, 2014, was the last day I did chemotherapy.

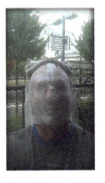

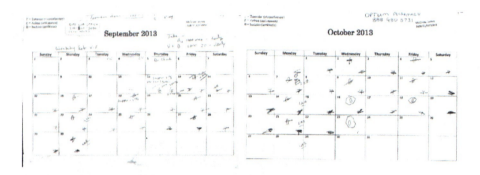

The two calendars above is when it hit home. I had cancer, a very serious cancer. I was going to die if I didn't do something. I started out listening to the Medical Staff. I figured they knew what to do. I found later the Doctor's, The Nurse's, Researcher's only know what they are taught. *Surgery, chemotherapy, and radiation* is *what they are taught.* They are so wrong. It is the worst way to treat cancer. The cancer industry is huge. It makes a lot of money and Big Pharma is not going to change that. They have everyone believing they are searching for a cure. Even the media believes they are looking for a cure.

I started doing research on the internet after I got to Memphis in November 2013. I am still doing research. It was in December 2013, and I was thinking about trying Cannabis Oil. I had heard that Cannabis Oil was the best thing for cancer. Back then it was extremely expensive. You could not get it in America. You had to go through Canada and use a Pay-Pal account. Who knows if was legitimate? I was not going to try.

As I was scrolling through the websites looking for Cannabis Oil. I came across this website that said, "Garlic Kills Brain Cancer Without Side Effects". This is the website. I did nothing but Garlic from December 2013 until December 2015
https://healthimpactnews.com/2014/garlic-kills-brain-cancer-cells-without-side-effects/?fbclid=IwAR2WcHddJlw0M1hF7StdsrMRYyjw9byk560x444yH_Ep8_CmrJ2pimn4K54
Jan 6, 2014, by DAVE MIHALOVIC

Garlic Kills Brain Cancer Cells Without Side Effects

- Health Impact News - https://healthimpactnews.com -
Garlic Kills Brain Cancer Cells Without Side Effects
Posted By *Site Admin* On January 9, 2014 @ 12:04 pm In Alternative Health

People on Facebook wanted me to write a book so I wrote an E-Book where I could edit it. Some of the Facebook people wanted a Paperback. I had to learn how to do a Paperback. It took a lot of time. I uploaded it from what I had written in Microsoft Word. It was disaster. The margins were off everything was off.

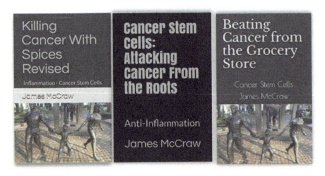

There was no Table of Contents. I did not know how easy it was to write a Table of Contents in Word. I ordered my book on Amazon and started reading. It was horrible. I did not proof-read it and there so many mistakes and where I would leave out words. (It is a cancer thing) I had to clean up the mistakes and the book was out already. I called the new book "Killing Cancer With Spices Revised" then I wrote "Cancer Stem Cells: Attacking Cancer From the Roots" and the latest book "Beating Cancer from the Grocery Store".

People were still going to do chemotherapy and radiation first. I have learned from honest Doctors that know chemotherapy and radiation therapy is absolutely the worst thing you can do. You must kill the **Cancer Stem Cells** and chemotherapy and radiation will not the **Cancer Stem Cells**. In this book I am going to highlight the things that you would not find at the grocery store. I am going to include what I did to beat cancer from the grocery store. So, you do not have to buy the previous books.

I have been using these 4 things, Garlic, Turmeric, Ginger and Cayenne Pepper to beat cancer. As of 2015 I am cancer free. The last I did chemotherapy was May 5, 2014. That is why I called my first book "Killing Cancer With Spices"

I added Cinnamon, Blueberry's, Strawberry's, Black Seed Oil, Honey, Coconut Oil, Extra Virgin Olive Oil, Avocado Oil. So, I wrote the book "**Beating Cancer from the Grocery Store**". Now I am going to show you how to beat cancer with cannabis oil, melatonin, high dosages of melatonin, and IP-6 and what I did to beat cancer.

Some are thinking if he didn't follow procedures of taking Garlic why didn't he stick with Garlic. If I was sure that Garlic killed the cancer I would stick with Garlic. Each thing I do fights cancer in a different way. **<u>Do not stick with one thing to beat cancer.</u>**

As time went on, I discovered some other things to beat cancer. I was already cancer free, but it could not hurt. I had already known about cannabis oil. I still have not tried cannabis oil. It is a good thing if you have cancer to add cannabis oil. I know a lot of people that tried it. Most of the ones that tried cannabis oil was cancer free. The cancer shrunk and then came back, and unfortunately, most of them died. I think it was that cancer found another way to bypass the cannabis oil. **<u>Do not stick with one thing to beat cancer.</u>** Typically, you only get one shot at beating cancer.

I added Melatonin and IP-6 in 2021 just because it was available and relatively cheap. I do not think I would need it, but you never know.

Glioblastoma Multiforme Grade 4 do not typically shrink, especially with no treatment whatsoever. As I said before, I had chemotherapy on May 5, 2014. It was last time I did chemotherapy. I did not use any sort of treatment. The only drug I did was Levetiracetam (Keppra), a non-seizure drug. It was sometime around May or June 2016 when the MRI showed that it was shrinking. That was about 2 years with no treatments. I did everything I could from the grocery store to fight cancer. The book 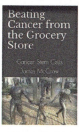 before this one was called "**Beating Cancer from the Grocery Store**" it is available on Amazon. You must eat so you might as well kill the **Cancer Stem Cells** while you are eating. It is about eating anti-inflammation because they kill the **Cancer Stem Cells**. Killing the **Cancer Stem Cells** is the target, not the tumor. The tumor is there to save your life. When your body is full of poison. If you kill the **Cancer Stem Cells**, then you can say you are cancer free. If you do not kill the **Cancer Stem Cells** the cancer will spread, it is called metastasis.

[Cancer stem cells, cancer cell plasticity and radiation therapy - PubMed (nih.gov)](#) "Since the first prospective identification of **cancer stem cells** in solid cancers the **cancer stem cell** hypothesis has reemerged as a research topic of increasing interest. It postulates that solid cancers are organized hierarchically with a small number of **cancer stem cells** driving tumor growth, repopulation after injury and *metastasis*. They give rise to differentiated progeny, which lack these features. The model predicts that for any therapy to provide cure, all **cancer stem cells** must be *eliminated* while the survival of differentiated progeny (tumor) is less critical. In this review we discuss recent reports challenging the idea of a unidirectional differentiation of cancer cells. These reports provide evidence supporting the idea that non-stem cancer cells exhibit a remarkable degree of plasticity that allows them to re-acquire **cancer stem cell** traits, especially in the context of radiation therapy. We summarize conditions under which differentiation is reversed and discuss the current knowledge of the underlying mechanism

My Journey

It all started at a café in Dallas on a Monday. I went to work, and something didn't feel right. I went to a café to eat and get some coffee. The next thing I know I had no use of my body, and I could not talk. I was just sitting there with my head leaning to the right and my head was shaking. I was awake but had no control. Finally, the waitress noticed me. I heard her say "He is having a seizure" The seizure ended about 5 minutes later. Someone had called the Paramedics and they

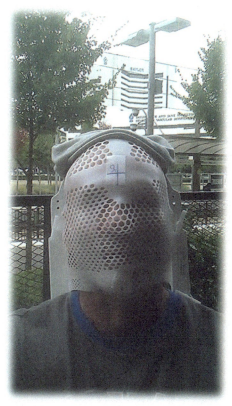

couldn't find anything wrong with me. They told me too just be careful. I called my girlfriend and she told me told I should go to a hospital right away. She would meet me at my apartment. Baylor Downtown was basically my backyard. She met me at my apartment, and we walked to the Baylor Emergency Room. It was not long after I was there that I had another seizure. Same as before, about 5 minutes long and I was awake during the seizure. They sent me for an MRI, and it turned out to be a brain tumor. I didn't panic I called my sister in Memphis and told her the news. I was determined to beat this. I didn't want to know the prognosis because I was determined to beat it. It was a Glioblastoma, but the Doctors could not tell if it was a level 3 or 4. The worst being a 4. The surgeon debated with his team on how to proceed. He could use a needle to get a sample of the tumor, or he could just wait until after the surgery and find out then. He chose to wait until after the surgery. I had to have an awake craniotomy. I had to be awake during part of it to make sure they didn't take too much and leave me a vegetable. The surgery was scheduled for August 13, 2013. I worked until the day before surgery. I think I remember being woke up or maybe it was a dream. The surgeon had told me beforehand that I wouldn't see him because he was behind me. I think I remember a few people in lab coats doing whatever they do in surgery. Most of the tumor was a Grade 3 but there was enough of it that was a Grade 4 that by the standards he was forced to call it a Grade 4. The surgery went well still no headaches. I felt fine. A couple of friends smuggled beer into the hospital room, and we had a party.

My cousin was the closest relative in Dallas. She took care of me, but she lived about 40 minutes north of Dallas. She helped me set up schedules and calendars so I would know when to take my chemo (Temodar) and other medicines. She was a lot of help, but she had a job and other things to take care of. The only person left was my Dad in Memphis. He came down but he wasn't much help, but it was nice of him to come to Dallas. I didn't know what to expect. Everyone had doom and gloom stories. My Oncologist and friends told it would get much worse and I was afraid of what would happen if Dad wasn't there. He was a real trooper. He is a diabetic and doesn't manage his insulin very well so he would go into low blood-sugar and become delirious so I wouldn't let him drive me around. He went into low blood-sugar a few times while he was staying with me. Our key phrase "Are you in your right mind" If he didn't answer I gave him orange juice and he snapped right back.

My loft was on the Light Rail Station. I could go out of my personal gate and be on the Dart Light Rail train station. I had to use the light rail system a lot. I would use it to fill my prescriptions, get groceries and anything else I wanted to do. Baylor Hospital was on the other side of the rail system.

On September 3rd, 2013, I began Rehab. It was from 9am-3pm. September 12, 2013, is when I started chemo for 42 straight days. It was 150 mg of Temodar. I would take it after my last meal. You had to stay vertical for 30 minutes after you took it. I would go for a walk, or to see a local band play, or the run on the treadmill. September 18, 2013, I started 30 days of radiation it ended October 29, 2013. It would last about 15 minutes Monday-Friday. I would walk home. I wish I would have known that there are alternate treatments available. I probably would have skipped the chemo and radiation and possibly the surgery.

I was going to move back to my hometown, Memphis Tennessee, but first I had to complete the first round of chemo, finish radiation and be released from rehab. It took until the middle of November 2013 before I was released from Baylor. The day finally came to be released from Baylor. I had already sold my car to my cousin, filed bankruptcy, and applied for Affordable Health Care (Obamacare) I started the process of moving my Baylor medical care from Dallas to Memphis before I left Dallas. This was stressful I could barely speak on the phone. A lot of calls started with a recording. Every time I would call it was it the same recording. I was trying to not become so stressed out. I applied to Obamacare too soon I should have waited till I moved from Dallas to Tennessee, and I was on Social Security Disability. I jumped the gun. Every time I'd call Obamacare, they would create another account. It was a mess. I was out of vacation time on August 27, 2013, so I had no income until Social Security Disability kicked in. My former employer gave me a going away gift. They were going to give me enough money that would cover Cobra for 1 ½ years. I paid Cobra for 6 months until I could get Obamacare straightened out. I had no long-term disability. I went to the mailbox one day and there was check, my Mom had died of Pancreatic Cancer a few years earlier. I signed up for a Cancer Policy that paid thousands of dollars so that was a huge relief.

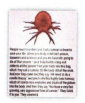

The Bottom Line - Kill the Cancer Stem Cells

The bottom line is you must kill the **Cancer Stem Cells (CSC)** The tumor is not the target the **Cancer Stem Cells** are the target. "People need to understand that a tumor is there to save your life. When your body is full of poison, and you are basically going to die of that poison - your body builds a bag and collects all the poison from your body into this bag, which they call a tumor."

It does not matter how you do it. There are many ways to kill the **Cancer Stem Cells**. There is cannabis oil, melatonin, high levels melatonin, IP-6, and metformin, and repurposed drugs

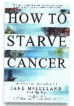

13

(Jane McClelland) wrote a book "**How To Starve Cancer**". The **Cancer Stem Cells (CSC)** are the mother of all cancers, all cancer starts with **Cancer Stem Cells**. The only way to be truthfully "cancer free" is to kill the **Cancer Stem Cells (CSC)**.

The Cancer Industry, like I said before, is huge. They are not too eager to let their cash-cow disappear until they can find a way to profit off the **Cancer Stem Cells**. The **Cancer Stem Cells** has been around since the 1990's. Big Pharma don't give two cents about you. Chemotherapy and radiation and surgery does not kill the **Cancer Stem Cells** and prescribing chemotherapy and radiation makes them a lot of money. How much do you pay for treatment? The Cancer Industry (Big Pharma and the FDA) does not teach the Doctors and Oncologists about the **Cancer Stem Cells** or **nutrition**. That is no excuse for being ignorant of the facts or too lazy. They only know what they are taught. Most of the Doctors and Oncologists are arrogant. There is a lot of information on **PubMed** about the **Cancer Stem Cells**. This is a resource the Doctors use. **The Cancer Stem Cells** have been around since the 1990's.

PubMed®

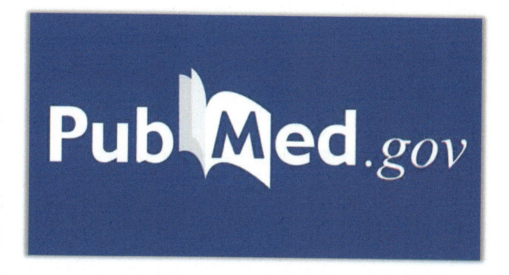

A service of the National Library of Medicine, PubMed® contains publication information and (in most cases) brief summaries of articles from scientific and medical journals. For guidance from NCCIH on using PubMed, see How To Find Information About Complementary Health Approaches on PubMed.
Website: https://pubmed.ncbi.nlm.nih.gov/
NIH Clinical Research Trials and You
The National Institutes of Health (NIH) has created a website, NIH Clinical Research Trials and You, to help people learn about clinical trials, why they matter, and how to participate. The site includes questions and answers about clinical trials, guidance on how to find clinical trials through ClinicalTrials.gov and other resources, and stories about the personal experiences of clinical trial participants.

Clinical trials are necessary to find better ways to prevent, diagnose, and treat diseases.
  Website: https://www.nih.gov/health-information/nih-clinical-research-trials-you
  National Heart, Lung, and Blood Institute (NHLBI)
  The NHLBI Health Information Center provides information to health professionals, patients, and the public about heart, lung, and blood diseases and sleep disorders and accepts orders for publications.
  P.O. Box 30105
  Bethesda, MD 20824-0105
  Toll-free in the U.S.: 1-877-NHLBI4U (1-877-645-2448)
  Website: https://www.nhlbi.nih.gov/
Email: nhlbiinfo@nhlbi.nih.gov

Do a search on: PubMed Cancer. And follow the links.

Do a search on: PubMed Cancer Stem Cells. Another list comes up.

Cancer stem cells: A brief review of the current status - PubMed (nih.gov)
Cancer stem cells (CSCs) comprise the subpopulation of tumor bulk and acquire resistant to conventional therapies and are considered as the primary tumor initiator cells. Nowadays, the tumor heterogeneity originated from CSCs, and its progenitors are accepted as a mortifying drawback in front of the cancer therapies. However, escalating knowledge gained from studies investigating the biology of CSCs will open up new frames for targeted therapies and decrease the chance of recurrence of the disease. In this review, the general understanding of CSCs and current studies were discussed briefly. Considering the latest data collected from studies of CSCs, defining the tumor heterogeneity and tumor microenvironment comprehensively will be very important to step up the cancer research.

[Cancer stem cell] - PubMed (nih.gov)
  Recently it is considered that there is a small population of cells with stem cell property not only in leukemia but also in solid cancer. These cells show the ability of **self-renewal** and multi-potential differentiation and can initiate and maintain a **tumor**. The origin of cancer stem cells might be their normal stem cells, progenitor cells, or bone marrow-derived cells. It is still difficult to isolate **cancer stem cells**

in solid cancer. There are three possible methodologies to isolate or identify cancer stem cells; the use of a surface marker, use of cells cultured in a specific condition (sphere), or the use of side population cells identified by FACS. The gold standard assay that fulfills the definition of **cancer stem cell** may be serial transplantation in animal models. **Cancer stem cells** are likely to be responsible for _disease relapse or metastasis_, and also for _resistance to radiation or conventional chemotherapy_. The stem cell niche plays an important role on maintaining **cancer stem cells**. The novel promising therapies against **cancer stem cells** are considered, including antibody-based therapy, signal inhibitors, overcoming radiation and drug resistance, or differentiation therapy. Another interesting therapy targeting the niche may also be considered.

Cancer stem cells, cancer cell plasticity and radiation therapy - PubMed (nih.gov)

Since the first prospective identification of cancer stem cells in solid cancers the **cancer stem cell** hypothesis has reemerged as a research topic of increasing interest. It postulates that solid cancers are organized hierarchically with a small number of **cancer stem cells** _driving tumor growth_, _repopulation after injury and metastasis_. They give rise to differentiated progeny, which lack these features. The model predicts that for any therapy to provide cure, all **cancer stem cells** _must be eliminated_ while the survival of differentiated progeny is less critical. In this review we discuss recent reports challenging the idea of a unidirectional differentiation of cancer cells. These reports provide evidence supporting the idea that non-stem cancer cells exhibit a remarkable degree of plasticity that allows them to re-acquire **cancer stem cell** traits, especially in the context of _radiation therapy_. We summarize conditions under which differentiation is reversed and discuss the current knowledge of the underlying mechanisms.

So, why is it, that a guy with no medical experience can find this? The Doctors are either lying or they are too lazy to find the truth.

Bharat B. Aggarwal, PhD

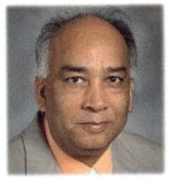

From Wikipedia, the free encyclopedia
I think Bharat Aggarwal is a genius and I give him credit for saving my life. I don't know what happened at the University of Texas MD Anderson Cancer Center. I have tried to email him to thank him. I can only assume but I think he was let go because he was about to blow the entire cancer research industry out of the water. He was on a Podcast called 'Power Hour' and he said cancer is all about inflammation. If you control your inflammation, you control cancer. He was one of the first to say everyone has cancer. You can't find a cure if everyone has cancer. The lady hosting the show said aren't you going get in trouble for being so honest in this interview. That is the last interview that I heard from Bharat.

https://www.youtube.com/watch?v=Zht2Q5D0RdY

Bharat B. Aggarwal PhD
From Wikipedia, the free encyclopedia

Bharat B. Aggarwal is an Indian American biochemist. His research has been in the areas of cytokines, the role of inflammation in cancer, and the anti-cancer effects of spices and herbs, particularly those of curcumin (a chemical constituent of the spice turmeric). He was a professor in the Department of Clinical Immunology, Bio immunotherapy, and Experimental Therapeutics at University of Texas MD Anderson Cancer Center in Houston, Texas, a position from which he retired in 2015 following allegations of fraud in his research.

He was formerly with M.D Anderson in Houston. Tx. He did not see eye to eye with a lot of the M.D Anderson staff. He is retired now. I think he was ahead of his time. He saved my life. He started looking at different cancers and he noticed that all cancers had one thing in common. There was inflammation in all the cancers he saw.

He also said it was a ***chronic*** disease and not a disease that can be ***cured***. He is probably the first one to notice this. He is of the opinion that cancer is caused by inflammation. The same as Diabetes, Arthritis, Psoriasis, Alzheimer's. If you can control inflammation, you can control all these diseases. I started eating foods that were anti-inflammatory. He was big on Curcumin. A byproduct of Turmeric. Turmeric only has about 4-5% of Curcumin. He also said everyone has cancer cells in their bodies. In some people it becomes a problem. That is another reason there is no cure for cancer. Bharat, as far as I know, never mentioned Cancer Stem Cells (CSC) As it turned out, everything I was eating was anti-inflammatory and killed the Cancer Stem Cells (CSC)

In 2012, MD Anderson launched a review of Aggarwal's research after the federal government notified them of allegations of fraud by academic whistleblowers in as many as 65 of Aggarwal's published papers, one of which had been retracted by the journal that published it. Several more of Aggarwal's publications were subsequently retracted after they were found to contain data images that had been reused and manipulated to represent different results. Aggarwal resigned from his position at MD Anderson at the end of 2015. By August 2016, eighteen research articles published by Aggarwal (in seven scientific journals) had been retracted.

I think the above ordeal was to discredit Doctor Aggarwal. The Cancer Industry (Big Pharma) is not going sit back and let the Cancer Industry implode. There is lot of money at stake and Aggarwal is telling people to watch their inflammation. He retired at the end of 2015. As of today, he is still fighting cancer and I am going 7 years in July 2020 being cancer free with a Glioblastoma Multiforme Grade 4 cancer.

Cancer is a chronic metabolic disease. Chronic diseases can be controlled, not cured. There is no cure for cancer

Doctor Bradford Weeks M.D.

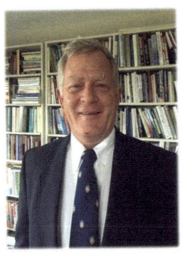

Years of Experience: 28
Specialties: Preventive medicine - public health & general preventive medicine · Psychiatry & neurology - psychiatry

<u>EXECUTIVE SUMMARY</u>

Dr. Weeks' medical license was **stolen** in 2013 because his practice of holistic or integrative medicine was deemed a "theoretical" risk of harm to the public. No patients were harmed, and no patients complained. The Washington State medical board (MQAC) has a track record to harassment of integrative medical doctors and the sanction which the medical board (MQAC) levied against Dr. Weeks was finally admitted by their counsel, almost 7 years after the fact, to be impossible to fulfill. That means Dr, Weeks has been suffering an illegal de facto revocation of his license to care for patients for 7 years. The administrative courts have not protected his constitutional rights, so Dr. Weeks is appealing now for donations to fund his appeal at a higher civil court which understands its obligation to protect the constitutional rights of all citizens.

https://weeksmd.com/2020/07/dr-weeks-and-cancer-stem-cells/

Dr. Weeks and Cancer STEM Cells
Dr. Gerber, President of Nevada Medical Society report of Dr. Weeks' lecture
Bradford S. Weeks, MD
CCC (Corrective Cancer Care), IPT (Insulin Potentiated Therapy), CSC (Cancer Stem Cells), QOL (Quality of Life) and the Cordelia Effect in the Treatment of People with Cancer

I (Dr Gerber) thought Dr. Weeks's lecture was truly revolutionary (www.weeksmd.com). A great student of medicine and literature, he is a fine wordsmith and communicator. In Shakespeare's King Lear, Lear's third daughter, Cordelia, proved to be the most beloved and loyal. Using this analogy to cancer therapy, Weeks unwinds the kinder, gentler, and more comprehensive approach to cancer care. He is an orthomolecular psychiatrist, rigorous researcher, humanitarian, musician, and apitherapist from Washington State, with extensive writing and international lecturing experience.

Cancer, he notes, is not the problem; cancer is an adaptive response to the problem. Toxic blood and tissue (the mesenchyme) is the problem.

Insulin Potentiated Therapy

The first IPT was used in 1946 by Donato Perez Garcia Sr., MD, to successfully treat breast cancer. Cancer cells have extensive insulin and IGF-1 receptors and have from 6 to 17 times more insulin receptors per cell than noncancer cells. Insulin targets cancer cells and enhances anticancer drug effects, which can be effective in much smaller doses than usual chemotherapy treatment. Only 2% of all cancers respond to traditional chemotherapy at the five-year survival level.9 Insulin enhanced the cytotoxic effect of methotrexate in MCF-7 human breast cancer cells in vitro by a factor of up to 10,000-fold.10

Glucose is the only fuel that cancer cells can use. Cancer cells have 10 times the IGF-1 receptors as regular cells.11 Insulin increases delta 9-desaturase, which makes cancer cells become permeable. IGF-1 doubles the number of cancer cells in S-phase: increasing vulnerability to chemotherapy drugs. Cancer cells are selectively targeted so that lower doses of chemotherapy can be used, which are highly effective and preserve immune function. It also increases appetite, weight, and euphoria.

Nutrients

Lifestyle, exercise, quality thoughts, and supplements are all part of Weeks's program for corrective cancer care. He notes that caffeine forces apoptosis, along with curcumin and turmeric. Theanine increases gamma interferon, arginine increases natural killer cells and T-cell function. American ginseng increases T-cell function, melatonin increases IL-2 and epidermal growth factor. Vitamins A, C, and D are also important along with aromatase inhibitors, BioDim, and Myomin. To prevent metastases, Weeks recommends modified citrus pectic, heparin, and thalidomide. Fermented soy in Haelan 951 contains isoflavones, protease inhibitors, saponins, phytosterols, and phytic acid compounds. Proteolytic enzymes taken away from food selectively attack and kill cancer cells, clean up debris, unmask cancer cells (membrane effect), prevent metastatic disease, and offer systemic immune enhancement with a compelling scientific, clinical record.

Vitamin D3 has 63 recent studies that have shown that the incidence of colon, breast, and ovarian cancer can be dramatically reduced by increasing the public's intake of vitamin D.12 Vitamin K3 especially in combination with vitamin C showed synergistic effects. High-dose IV vitamin C infusions have been shown to have cytotoxic effects in most cancer cell lines in vitro. The mechanism appears to be intracellular accumulation of H2O2 with low catalase enzyme activity native to cancer cells. Vitamin C has also been found to potentiate the effects of chemotherapy drugs.13

Cancer Stem Cells
Max Wicha, MD, distinguished professor of oncology and director of the University of Michigan Comprehensive Cancer Center, has delivered a startling revelation that standard cancer treatments not only often fail to eradicate cancer, but they can make it worse. The reason that breast cancer and other malignancies often return aggressively after treatment is that when tumor cells die under assault from chemotherapy and radiation, they give off substances that can reactivate a special set of master cells known as cancer stem cells. Dr. Wicha's lab has found that inflammatory molecules secreted by dying tumor cells (IL-8) can hook up with the stem cells and cause them in effect to come out of hibernation. Cancer stem cells are relatively resistant to cytotoxic chemotherapeutics and radiation. "Chemotherapy and radiation make cancer worse."

Dr. Weeks offers many treatments to help suppress **cancer stem cells**. Please get his entire lecture from NHIMA; and he had a lecture scheduled at the Orthomolecular Health Medicine conference February 24, 2012, in San Francisco. He thinks that it is necessary to reeducate confused cancer stem cells by changing the body's environment with anti-inflammatory agents to disrupt the IL-8 cytokine "SOS" and allow differentiation of cancer stem cells. Such agents include Reprotaxin, a cancer cell receptor 1 blocker (per Dr. Wicha), soy, above nutrients, and enzymes, as well as iodine (iodolactones), which increased apoptosis in 80% of breast cancer cell lines.

High on Fermented Soy
Haelan 951 is a potent treatment for cancer that decreases pro-inflammatory cytokines including IL8 and promotes cell differentiation in five cancer cell lines in vitro, as shown in studies dating from 1990.16 This fermented soy product also promotes antiangiogenesis and stem cell metastasis by its anti-inflammatory mechanism. It improves apoptosis of cancer cells, and DNA repair, reactivates P-53 tumor suppressor gene, and increases P21 activity. It also reduces estrogen levels,

increases estrogen receptor-beta receptors (ER-b), decreases estrogen receptor-alpha (ER-a), and decreases matrix metalloproteinase enzymes, which erode collagen containment of tumor cells and allow cancer stem cells to spread throughout the body, creating metastases. This product also helps prevent protein calories malnutrition (cachexia or starvation), which kills 80% of cancer patients. It shuts down that NF-kB mutation pathway, which is used by cancer cells to escape death, and enhances tumor necrosis factor (TNF), a pillar of our immune system required to fight cancer. Fermented soy overcomes depression with improved quality of life and increases nonspecific immune stimulation by 400%, with macrophage levels improving 3-fold, and doubles the number of active macrophages. Other positive characteristics include reduction of exosomes, which are particles that inhibit both NK cells and gamma interferon and increasing BAX gene 500% that kills cancer cells via allowing *apoptosis* and decreasing BCL2 gene by 200%, which allows cancer cells to thrive by evading apoptosis.

Taking Haelan fermented soy 4 oz twice per day may be challenging in regard to taste; it is very bitter. Weeks recommends taking it with stevia/xylitol and Ola Loa Orange drink, one packet in cold water. It may also be taken via retention enema.

Metformin for CSC

New data from Cancer Research Journal 2011 in May demonstrate that metformin selectively kills chemotherapy-resistant cancer stem cells in breast cancer cell lines, and studies in Medical Oncology February 2011 suggest several mechanisms for its ability to suppress cancer growth in vitro and vivo.17,18 It activates LKB1/AMPK pathway, induction of cell cycle arrest and/or apoptosis, inhibits protein synthesis, reduces insulin levels, inhibits the unfolded protein response, activates the immune system, and eradicates cancer stem cells.

Summary: Stem Cells and Cancer

"Cancer mortality is directly related to cancer stem cell activity (metastatic and proliferative processes). **Chemotherapy and radiation do not kill cancer stem cells**. Chemotherapy and radiation make cancers grow faster and more virulently. Treatment of cancer patients requires adjunctive care. Treatment which fails to address the toxicity of **cancer stem cells** is futile and irresponsible". Please go online to Dr. Weeks's websites to get all of the citations for further reading on stem cell treatments and leading researchers in the field, including Walter Wainright (Haelan Research Foundation); **Max Wicha, MD**; Michael Clark, MD, director, Stanford Institute for Stem Cell and Regenerative Medicine; Max Diehn, MD, oncology radiologist, Stanford University; and Ursula Jacob, MD.

Clinical Case Studies

Dr. Weeks presents five clinical case studies with phenomenal outcomes. Stage 4 cancers with a death sentence responded to his therapies with great success. Please read his full reports from his lecture on NHIMA DVDs or from his website. In addition to the above treatments, he uses LDN 4.5 mg, low-dose naltrexone touted to stop tumor growth. Cimetidine is also added for its antitumor effect. He uses chemosensitivity testing via Biofocus in Germany, which grows cancer cells in culture and determines which chemotherapy and nutrient therapies induce apoptosis and focus on which chemotherapeutic agents are most effective in IPT. In addition, he uses IV vitamin C 50 to 75 g backed by alpha-lipoic acid 600 mg by IV push 3 hours later to improve the oxidative stress on cancer cells by vitamin C. (Thanks to Bert Berkson, MD, who has championed alpha-lipoic acid for many decades.) Weeks also uses homeopathic and anthroposophical remedies such as aurum stibium, Hyoscyamus, hepar stannum, Lien cichorium, lymphocytes 8, thrombocytes 6, and erythrocytes 6. In addition to Haelan 951, Ioderal, multivitamin and mineral supplements, niacin, selenium, CoQ10, vitamin D3, LDN 4.5 mg, and metformin 500 mg b.i.d.

Doctor Weeks has a video online from The Truth About Cancer Symposium sponsored by Ty and Charlene Bollinger. It is a video about Cancer Stem Cells. He said, "chemotherapy and radiation will make your cancer worse" and attributed it to Max Wicha. I think Max is the guru of cancers. Doctor Weeks talks about chronic inflammation being a prime reason for cancer. He talks about cheap anti-inflammatory agents (I get my anti-Inflammatory agents from the grocery store you will see later in this book) In the video he has a slide that I found alarming "The Federation of State Medical Boards, CDC, FDA, AMA, Big Pharma all members of Corporate Medicine(i.e. the Medical Industrial Complex) are complicit in putting profit above patient health and wellness" he also mentions "The Standard of Care is oppressive and innovators lose their license" you can see the video at:

https://www.youtube.com/watch?time_continue=1023&v=MZKpGZMxMTE&feature=emb_logo

Max Wicha

Dr. Max S. Wicha
Internal medicine - medical oncology
Years of Experience: 44

Dr. Max S Wicha specializes in medical oncology in Ann Arbor, MI and has over 46 years of experience in the field of medicine. He graduated from Stanford University School Of Medicine with his medical degree in 1974. He is affiliated with numerous hospitals in Michigan and more, including University Of Michigan Health System. Dr. Max S Wicha is licensed to practice by the state board in Michigan (4301042541).

Max Wicha, M.D, the founder and director emeritus of the **University of Michigan**'s **Comprehensive Cancer Center**, has received a grant of $6.5 million from the **National Cancer Institute** to continue his research into *cancer stem cells*, the cells in a tumor that fuel its growth and its spread.

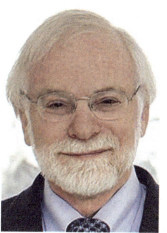

The award is about three times a traditional award for an individual investigator and is part of a new NCI grant program called R-35, which funds projects of unusual potential in cancer research over a period of seven years.

The goal is to give investigators enough time and support to break new ground or extend previous discoveries.

"With this kind of research, you don't always know where it's going next. This new grant gives us the freedom to pursue new directions in cancer stem cell research," said Wicha, the Madeline and Sidney Forbes Professor of Oncology at UM, in a press release.

Wicha has successfully commercialized his research in the past. He is the co-founder of Redwood City, Calif.-based **OncoMed Pharmaceuticals**, a biotechnology company that develops cancer treatments. He also has more than a dozen patents.

"The NCI Outstanding Investigator Award addresses a problem that many cancers researchers experience: finding a balance between focusing on their science while ensuring that they will have funds to continue their research in the future," said Dinah Singer, director of NCI's Division of Cancer Biology.

Wicha is one of the world's foremost ***cancer stem cell*** researchers and was part of the team that first identified stem cells in breast cancer, which was the first time they had been described in a solid tumor.

That has led to multiple clinical trials testing therapies aimed at attacking ***cancer stem cells***.

Wicha plans to use the grant to isolate circulating tumor cells, cancer cells that break off from the primary tumor and circulate throughout a patient's bloodstream.

Using devices developed by engineering colleagues, the team will isolate and analyze the genome of individual cancer cells and determined whether treatment is attacking the stem cells.

Wicha's lab will also work with other researchers understand the role the immune system plays in ***cancer stem cells***.

It Make Sense: Anti-Inflammatory and Cancer Stem Cells

Cancer is a chronic metabolic disease. Chronic diseases can be controlled, not cured. There is no cure for cancer the tumor is not the target. The Cancer Stem cells are the target

I came to reason that if you eat things that are not inflammatory (**anti-inflammatory**) to beat, **not cure**, cancer then maybe they are killing the **Cancer Stem Cells (CSC)**. I was right. I was on to something. Most, if not, all the anti-inflammatory foods also kill the *Cancer Stem Cells* (**CSC**). Take whatever internet browser you use and type in **"what foods kill the Cancer Stem Cells"**

I do not consider it as "My Protocol" or even as "my diet" It is the things you are supposed to eat. I hate it when people call it "My Protocol"

At first, I did not understand how the anti-inflammatory diet and the cancer stem cells were related. Everything I do to fight cancer also fights the Cancer Stem Cells. That is, in my opinion, the key to beating cancer. You must kill the *Cancer Stem Cells* to beat cancer. I have been told by many Doctors and Researchers that chemotherapy and radiation will not kill the Cancer Stem Cells. They can shrink the tumors but that is not the target. The Cancer Stem Cells is the target. Chemotherapy and Radiation, from I have been told, can make the cancer metastasize. That means the cancer can spread to other body parts. Killing the Cancer Stem Cells will not make it metastasize.

If you kill the **Cancer Stem Cells,** it does not matter what kind of cancer it is. You are killing the daughter cells before they develop into other cancer cells. Cancer cells are cells that divide relentlessly, forming solid tumors or flooding the blood with abnormal cells. Cell division is a normal process used by the body for growth and repair. A parent cell divides to form two daughter cells, and these daughter cells are used to build new tissue, or to replace cells that have died because of aging or damage. Healthy cells stop dividing when there is no longer a need for more daughter cells, but cancer cells continue to produce copies. They are also able to spread from one part of the body to another in a process known as **metastasis**. The Cancer Stem Cells (CSC) is the Mother of all cancers. The cancer that has already formed degenerates or regresses to nothing. If you kill the Cancer Stem Cells (CSC) you not only kill the CSC's but cancer in general. It does not matter what kind of cancer. It does not matter if it is an IDH-1 or what is DNA methylation. You are killing the Mother of all cancer before it gets the chance to be methylated.

Cancer Stem Cells (CSCs) have recently been identified in several solid tumors, including Brain, Breast, Colon, Head and Neck, Liver, Lung, Ovary, Pancreas, Prostate, Melanoma, Multiple Myeloma, Non-melanoma skin cancer, Stomach

This a brief excerpt from lengthy topic. I just wanted to see how important of killing the **Cancer Stem Cells (CSC)**

https://www.ncbi.nlm.nih.gov/pmc/articles/PMC4620424/

Traditional therapies against cancer, chemo- and radiotherapy, have multiple limitations that lead to treatment failure and cancer recurrence. These limitations are related to systemic and local toxicity, while treatment failure and cancer relapse are due to drug resistance and self-renewal, properties of a small population of tumor cells called **cancer stem cells (CSCs)**. These cells are involved in cancer initiation, maintenance, metastasis, and recurrence. Therefore, in to develop efficient treatments that can induce a long-lasting clinical response preventing tumor relapse it is important to develop drugs that can specifically target and eliminate **CSCs**. Recent identification of surface markers and understanding of molecular feature associated with **CSC** phenotype helped with the design of effective treatments. In this review we discuss targeting surface biomarkers, signaling pathways that regulate **CSCs** self-renewal and differentiation, drug-efflux pumps involved in *apoptosis* resistance, microenvironmental signals that sustain **CSCs** growth, manipulation of miRNA expression, and induction of **CSCs** *apoptosis* and differentiation, with specific aim to hamper **CSCs** regeneration and cancer relapse. Some of these agents are under evaluation in preclinical and clinical studies, most of them for using in combination with traditional therapies. The combined therapy using conventional anticancer drugs with CSCs-targeting agents, may offer a promising strategy for management and eradication of different types of cancers.

Core tip: **Cancer stem cells (CSCs)** play important roles in tumor formation, metastasis, and cancer relapse. In this article, we review the literature on the recent progress in developing anti-cancer stem cell strategies based on improved understanding of **CSCs** properties and molecular features. These novel therapeutic systems are designed with the aim of eradicating **CSCs,** by targeting surface specific markers and altering signaling pathways or mechanisms involved in **CSCs** maintenance and drug resistance, and also to disturb microenvironmental signals that sustain CSCs growth, with specific aim of impede **CSCs** regeneration and cancer relapse.

$$$The Bottom Line $$$

People need to understand that a **tumor** is there to save your life. When your body is full of poison, and you are basically going to die of that poison - your body builds a bag and collects all the poison from your body into this bag, which they call a **tumor**. The bottom line is you must kill the Cancer Stem Cells (CSC).

It does not matter how you do it. There are many ways I am just showing you what I do. The Cancer Stem Cells (CSC) is the Mother of cancer, all cancer starts with Cancer Stem Cells. The only way to be truthfully "cancer free" is to kill the Cancer Stem Cells (CSC). I am beginning to sound like a broken record (that is a 70's reference)

The Cancer Industry, like I said before, is huge. They are not too eager to let their cash-cow disappear until they can find a way to profit off the Cancer Stem Cells. Just try and imagine how big it is. They don't give two cents about you. Chemotherapy and radiation and all the other stuff they prescribe makes them a lot of money. How much do you pay for treatment?

For Chemotherapy and Radiation
Chemotherapy - $$$$$$
Radiation - $$$$$$

- They do not kill the Cancer Stem Cells

Compare that to:
Organic Garlic – $3.99 lb.
Organic Turmeric - $8.30 lb.
Organic Ginger - $13.59 lb.
Organic Cayenne Pepper – $3.99 1.69 oz.
Organic Blueberries - $5.99 half pint
Organic Strawberries - $4.99 lb.
Organic Avocados - $1.99 ea.
Organic Bananas - $0.69 lb.
Organic Green Bell Pepper - $2.49 lb.
Ceylon Cinnamon - $4.99
Organic Almond Butter - $10.99 16 oz
Black Seed Oil - $30.99 8 oz
Local Honey - $10.79 24oz

- They all kill the Cancer Stem Cells
- They are all anti-inflammatory

What Happens If You Don't' Kill the Cancer Stem Cells

https://www.ncbi.nlm.nih.gov/pmc/articles/PMC5523038/figure/fig01/

The following diagram is a list of 4 things that will happen when you have cancer. It is the best diagram I that have ever seen. If it does not grab your attention, then I do not know what will.

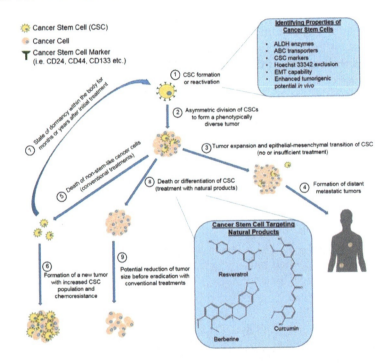

Illustration of the Cancer Stem Cell Model's explanation for tumor formation, metastasis, and recurrence and the potential of natural products in their treatment. Cancer Stem Cells (CSCs) are either formed upon carcinogenesis of somatic cells or stem cells, or they are activated after a period of dormancy (1). These CSCs then asymmetrically divide resulting in a phenotypically diverse tumor consisting of both CSCs and non-stem-like cells (2). Left untreated, the tumor will continue to grow and invade the surrounding tissue, and CSCs undergoing EMT may break off from the original tumor and travel to distant organs (3). The CSCs which reattach throughout the body can then initiate a new tumor, resulting in metastases (4). Using current treatment methods capable of inducing cell death in the bulk of tumor cells, the CSCs are not destroyed due to their enhanced survival traits, such as quiescence and the expression of ALDH enzymes and ABC transporters (5). The remaining CSCs may then go on to recreate the original tumor, sometimes increasing the percentage of CSCs within the tumor and forming multiple drug resistant tumors (6). In other cases, the remaining CSCs will enter a state of dormancy within the body and remain undetected for long periods of time before reactivating and initiating the formation of a new tumor, thus resulting in cancer relapse in patients thought to be cancer free. As a result of these issues, new treatments are being investigated which can target CSCs. Natural products have shown the potential to induce cell death in CSCs, cause CSCs to differentiate, or sensitize CSCs to conventional chemotherapy treatments, Once the CSCs have been eliminated, the remaining tumor may diminish in size and can be subsequently eradicated through the use of conventional antineoplastic therapies.

What I get out of this is there are 3 possibilities when you have cancer two are bad:
1) Killing the Cancer Stem Cells
2) Using Conventional Treatments
3) No or insufficient treatments

The first one, Number 1, is the way to go. Number 2 and 3 is not the way to go.

The only way I can see chemotherapy and radiation being used if it is an emergency like the tumor was getting too large and was intruding other body parts or cutting an airwave off.

Reactive vs Proactive

As far as I know there is 1 way to beat cancer. Kill the Cancer Stem Cells. Another way is the reactive way, or the conventional cancer treatment, (Chemotherapy and Radiation) where you get cancer and try the conventional cancer therapy for that particular cancer. Usually it is surgery, chemotherapy, and radiation. In each case it depends on where the cancer is if the cancer is IDH-1 or what kind of DNA methylation it is to determine what kind of chemotherapy or radiation. The cancer will Metastasize. Chemotherapy and radiation does shrink the tumor, but it stops when it gets to the Cancer Stem Cells (CSC) which is about 1% of tumor. The Oncologist gets excited and thinks it is a good thing, but it is not a good thing. That is the reactive way.

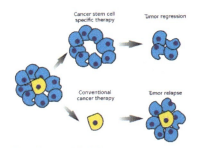

Peter Znamenskiy 1 Diagram

The other way, the one I prefer to beat cancer, is the **_proactive_** way, when you kill the Cancer Stem Cells (CSC). The tumor loses ability to generate new cells and tumor degenerates. You must kill the cancer from the **_roots_** and not from the top. If you chop your weeds and do not go down to the roots the weeds will grow back. It is the same way with cancer. The daughter cells are roots of all cancers. They are produced by the Cancer Stem Cells (CSC)

This method of killing the Cancer Stem Cells (CSC) kills pretty much all cancer including including: Brain, Breast, Colon, Head and Neck, Liver, Lung, Ovary, Pancreas, Prostate, Melanoma, Multiple Myeloma, Non-melanoma skin cancer, Stomach

As I said in a previous chapter. The Cancer Stem Cells (CSC) is the Mother of all cancers. The cancer that has already formed degenerates or regresses to nothing. If you kill the Cancer Stem Cells (CSC) you not only kill the CSC's but cancer in general. It does not matter what kind of cancer. People asks me if I am IDH-1 or what is my DNA methylation. If you kill the Cancer Stem Cells, it does not matter if it is IDH-1 or DNA methylation. That is ***reactive*** way of killing cancer. It does not matter if the cancer is methylated or not. You are killing the Mother of all cancer before it gets the chance to be methylated.

Falling into the Trap: Pharmaceutical vs Natural Products

Just about everything I do at breakfast kills the Cancer Stem Cells. Garlic, turmeric/curcumin, ginger, cayenne pepper, black seed oil, honey, cinnamon, pepper, strawberries, blueberries all kill the Cancer Stem Cells (CSC). I have a YouTube video that shows what I do every morning:
The YouTube link is: https://youtu.be/7KepWek8SSc

If you do not kill the Cancer Stem Cells (CSC) the cancer is most likely going to metastasize. It might not be immediately, but it will metastasize. Why is it that the Cancer Stem Cells (CSC) have been around since the 1990's but nobody seems to know about Cancer Stem Cells? Why did I happen to stumble across it 30 years later? Why are the Doctors still using chemotherapy and radiation to fight cancer? Did they miss the part where chemotherapy and radiation are bad and makes the cancer to metastasize? Maybe some are not taught that way and too lazy or too arrogant to research it.

The Doctors, Oncologist, Nurses, Researchers, Media, and you have fallen into this trap. Doctor Aggarwal said it has been going on for 50 years and he hopes it will not be 50 years to correct it. We need to stop with the Pharmaceutical Drugs and go back to Natural Products. A lot of Oncologist thinks that shrinking the tumor is good thing. That is not true. It is the opposite. The real target is the Cancer Stem Cells (CSC) The Cancer Stem Cells are only about 1%-3%. The Traditional Cancer Therapy (chemotherapy and radiation) will **_not_** kill the Cancer Stem Cells (CSC). In fact, they make it metastasize

Are There Other Ways to Kill Cancer Stem Cells?

If the **Cancer Stem Cell** theory is right, and if the killing the Cancer Stem Cells is the key to beating cancer. What is the best way to kill the Cancer Stem Cells? The Keto Diet, Cannabis Oil, Anti-Inflammation, These are all fall into the term anti-inflammation. Melatonin, IP-6, Metformin. I personally have not tried The Keto Diet or Cannabis Oil. I have recently tried Melatonin and IP-6 as of April 2021. Off label drugs that can fight cancer. See the book that Jane Mclellend wrote "How To Starve Cancer".

Another good cancer source is Chris Wark. He is a former cancer patient who refused chemotherapy. He is a tremendous source about cancer. He is NOT impressed with Big Pharma. He wrote books and podcasts. His webpage is https://www.chrisbeatcancer.com/

If you are wanting to beat cancer, try everything you can. "Don't put all your eggs in one basket" I know a lot of people that have tried one or two things and they are not here anymore. Try everything you can possibly do. I would try cannabis oil if I could afford it. The Keto Diet I am loosely following it. I do mean loosely, a lot of things I do would not fit in The Keto Diet. When I shop, I look at the carbs not the calories. You typically get one chance to beat cancer. For some it can be more but that is unlikely.

The Keto Diet

I have never tried The Keto Diet. I know some people had a lot of success with it. There are those that did not. I do about 50-75% of the Keto Diet. I personally don't think it is healthy or sustainable to stay in Ketosis. Some people would disagree. I do not think you can put your eggs in one basket. If you try The Keto Diet and that is up you, I think you are flirting with disaster. Cancer can find multiple pathways. You can shut down cancer in one, but it can find another pathway.

I did the **Atkin's Diet** in the 90's. The **Atkins Diet** is divided into different steps. The first step you do is they put you in **Ketosis**. The Atkin's Diet does not want you to stay in **Ketosis** for a long time. They don't believe it is healthy. I believe it is a couple of weeks. I did the Atkin's Diet too lose weight. I still am doing it. I count carbs and not calories. The goal is to find out how many carbs where you don't gain or lose any weight. Everybody has a different amount of carbs they can handle. Mine is about 80-100 carbs. That is the average.

You must cut bread out in the Keto Diet. Does that mean the only thing that can keep your sandwich together is lettuce? I tried it. It does not work for me. I do not think that all breads are a problem. I eat **Ezekiel Bread** I know it is good. The FDA gives a lot slack for what the breads can claim. For example: they can claim that it is **100% Wheat Bread** but is not. I did a chapter about bread in this book. You can go there to learn what kinds of bread is bad for you.

Cannabis Oil/CBD
https://theuniversalplant.com/cbd-inflammation/

In this post I am going to outline the collective body of current research on CBD and Hemp Extract with relation to Inflammation. There is a decent amount of research to this point, all indicating impressive benefits of CBD for inflammation, typically looking at inflammation biomarkers (indicators) and positive improvements when subjects use CBD or Hemp Extract over the control groups. CBD oil for inflammation is becoming increasingly more common as awareness around cannabis increases.

Melatonin

I started doing Melatonin and IP-6 just as a backup in 2021. I have been cancer free since 2014. I am taking 40 MG of Melatonin. I have heard people take 0.1 – 200 MG. Melatonin is produced by the pineal gland. Melatonin has showed that it can prompt apoptosis (cell suicide, programmed cell death) and inhibit tumor

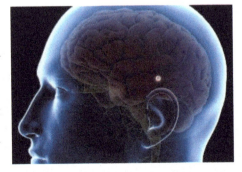

metastasis is such as ovarian, melanoma, colon, and breast cancer. It can kill the **Cancer Stem Cells** which it is
all about. It crosses the blood-brain barrier.

Tips To Consider
- Remember that even though the FDA regulates dietary supplements, such as melatonin, the regulations for dietary supplements are different and less strict than those for prescription or over-the-counter drugs.
- Some dietary supplements may interact with medicines or pose risks if you have medical problems or are going to have surgery.
- If you're pregnant or nursing a child, it's especially important to see your health care provider before taking any medicine or supplement, including melatonin.
- If you use dietary supplements, such as melatonin, read and follow label instructions. "Natural" doesn't always mean "safe." For more information, see Using Dietary Supplements Wisely.
- Take charge of your health—talk with your health care providers about any complementary health approaches you use. Together, you can make shared, well-informed decisions.

For More Information
NCCIH Clearinghouse

Targeting Cancer Stem Cells by Melatonin

This is a very important part of melatonin. I had no idea it could beat cancer and cause it to go into **apoptosis** (also called *cell suicide, programmed cell death*). Why is this not a headline in the news. I will use it in to beat cancer.

Effective therapy for cancer treatment
https://pubmed.ncbi.nlm.nih.gov/32171553/

Melatonin is a physiological hormone produced by the pineal gland. In recent decades, enormous investigations showed that melatonin can prompt **apoptosis** (also called *cell suicide, programmed cell death*) in **cancer** cells and inhibit tumor **metastasis** and angiogenesis in variety of malignancies such as ovarian, melanoma, colon, and breast cancer; therefore, its possible therapeutic usage in cancer treatment was confirmed. **Cancer Stem Cells**, which has received much attention from researchers in past decades, are major challenges in the treatment of cancer. Because **Cancer Stem Cells** are resistant to chemotherapeutic drugs and cause recurrence of cancer and have the ability to be regenerated; they can cause serious problems in the treatment of various cancers. For these reasons, the researchers are trying to find a solution to destroy these cells within the tumor mass. In recent years, the effect of **melatonin** on **Cancer Stem Cells** has been investigated in some cancers. Given the importance of **Cancer Stem Cells** in the process of cancer treatment, this article reviewed the studies conducted on the effect of **melatonin** on **Cancer Stem Cells** as a solution to the problems caused by **Cancer Stem Cells** in the treatment of various cancers.

High Dosages Melatonin

This is beyond me. I will let M.D., Ph.D., Jesus Tresquerres explain how High Dosages Melatonin can beat can cancer. I have not tried it. Experimental studies performed over more than 20 years have shown that oxidative stress and **inflammation** increase in nearly all tissues with many degenerative diseases or aging. We have measured several parameters related to oxidative stress, **inflammation, and apoptosis** both in several models of aging and after ischemia in the liver or brain. The effect of treatment with melatonin has been evaluated showing a significant reduction of **inflammation, apoptosis** markers and parameters related to oxidative stress, in several tissues. **Inflammations**, as well as oxidative stress and **apoptosis** markers were increased also in degenerative diseases like diabetes, hypertension, or Parkinson disease so treatment with melatonin should also have very positive effects.

Dosing

- Only red lights in the bedroom.
- Prevention: 180 mg about 30 minutes before bedtime.
- Treatment: 60 mg 3-6x/day
- 300mg two hours before PET/CT
- Melatonin Max – 60 mg pure capsules (www.scientifichealthsolutions.com)
- **Melatonin powder –** www.purebulk.com

Zero contraindications

IP-6

A friend of mine, Roger, told me about IP-6 in a coffee shop. I have been taking IP-6 since the spring of 2021. I get IP-6 on Amazon. That is the only place I found it.

Dosing:
- Most common anticancer dosage: 2-4 grams/day
- Anxiety and depression dosage: 12-18 grams/day

Precautions:
- IP6 has anti-platelet activity, so it may increase the risk of bleeding when used with other anticoagulants or anti-platelet drugs.
- IP6 can also bind with calcium, iron, magnesium, and zinc in the stomach and reduce their absorption.
- As always, discuss your use of any supplement with your physicians before taking them.

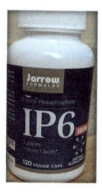

Animal and cell studies have reported that IP6 is effective in cancer prevention and control of tumor growth, progression, and metastasis. Its activity likely involves IP6's immune stimulatory, potent antioxidant and antiangiogenic effects.

Researchers have also discovered that when IP6 is combined with inositol, there is a significant synergistic effect against a variety of cancer types in cell and animal studies (i.e., colon, breast, lung, etc.) that far exceeds the anticancer activity of the individual compounds alone.

IP-6: Overview, Uses, Side Effects, Precautions, Interactions, Dosing and Reviews (webmd.com)

IP-6, inositol hexaphosphate, is a vitamin-like substance. It is found in humans, animals, and many plants, especially cereals, nuts, and legumes. It can also be made in a laboratory.

Some people use IP-6 to treat and prevent cancer, to reduce side effects of cancer treatment, for anemia, diabetes, and many other conditions, but there is no good scientific evidence to support these uses.

In manufacturing, IP-6 is added to food to keep it from spoiling.

How does it work ?

IP-6 might help treat and prevent cancer by slowing down the production of cancer cells. It might also bind to certain minerals, decreasing the risk of colon cancer. IP-6 is also an antioxidant.

Metformin

Metformin is something that I have never tried. It is supposedly a potential cancer fighting drug.

Metformin is well-known as an anti-diabetic drug, but it seems to possess anti-cancerous properties as well. Metformin's anti-cancerous properties have been demonstrated in various cancer cells in vitro, such as lung, pancreatic, colon, ovarian, breast, prostate, renal cancer cells, melanoma, and even in acute lymphoblastic leukemia cells. Metformin alone had no effect, and doxorubicin as a single agent initially shrank tumors, but they regrew later. **Virtually no cancer stem cells were recovered immediately after treatment and the complete response was sustained for nearly two months.** Although the results of recent trials confirm the efficacy of metformin in prevention and treatment of different cancers, the evidence are not adequate enough.

Inflammation to be Avoided

Sugar

Sugar is the Number 1 cause of **Inflammation.** You need to stop using sugar. Stop drinking sugary drinks. Stop soft drinks, including diet drinks. I heard aspartame is a big no-no and now Splenda is questionable so why not give it up. I drink water, unsweet tea, carrot juice, unsweetened green tea, almond milk, 1 or 2 cups of black coffee, for those cannot drink it black a little Half and Half or honey is okay. I could not make it through the day without 1 or 2 cups of coffee a day.

Cancer feeds on sugar? That question is asked all the time. Most Doctors either say no or say there is no definitive answer to that question. I say most definitely yes.

Many Doctors feel that cancer feeds on carbs and sugar. I do not use sugar or sugar alternates in anything. There is a smoothie that I drink every night that has 1 tablespoon of honey in it. **Honey works in reverse of sugar. Honey is good for fighting cancer.** If I get hungry for sweets. I use the low sugar candy bars. Honey, Sugar alcohol and Dietary Fiber are fine. If it is loaded with sugar stay away.

I started the Atkins Diet in 2003. It is a low-carb diet. To this day I look at the carbs and not the calories. If it has too many carbs, I do not buy it.

I buy non-dairy Yogurt with 7 grams of sugar or less. I found some Yogurt with no sugar in it. Keep your sugar in-take to a minimum. Before you know it, you are getting too much sugar just from the things you buy normally. Do not add to it by eating junk foods and processed foods.

<u>**Sugar alcohols**</u> (also called **polyhydric alcohols, polyalcohols, alditols** or **glycitols**) are organic compounds, typically derived from sugars, that comprise a class of polyols. They are white, water-soluble solids that can occur naturally or be produced industrially from sugars. They are used widely in the food industry as thickeners and sweeteners. In commercial foodstuffs, sugar alcohols are commonly used in place of table sugar (sucrose), often in combination with high intensity artificial sweeteners to counter the low sweetness. Xylitol and sorbitol are popular sugar alcohols in commercial foods.

https://theconsciouslife.com/top-10-inflammatory-foods-to-avoid.htm

Sugars

Sugar-sweetened beverages like soft drinks, fruit drinks and punches are some of the major sources of dietary sugars that many have overlooked. Do you know that drinking a can of Coke is as good as sucking ten sugar cubes? Other obvious sugar-loaded foods to avoid or at least limit include pastries, desserts, candies, and snacks. And when you are looking out for sugar in the ingredients list, note that sugar has many names: corn syrup, dextrose, fructose, golden syrup, maltose, sorghum syrup and sucrose are some of the creative names used.

Common Cooking Oils

Common vegetable cooking oils used in many homes and restaurants have very high omega-6 fatty acids and dismally low omega-3 fats. A diet consisting of a highly imbalanced omega-6 to omega-3 ratio promotes inflammation and breeds inflammatory diseases like heart disease and cancer.

Find them in: Polyunsaturated vegetable oils such as grape seed, cottonseed, safflower, corn, and sunflower oils. These industrial vegetable oils are also commonly used to prepare most processed foods and takeaways.

Trans Fats

Trans fatty acids are notorious for their double whammy effect: they increase the levels of 'bad' cholesterol, while lowering levels of the 'good' cholesterol. But that is not all they can do. They have also been found to promote inflammation, obesity, and resistance to insulin, laying the ground for degenerative illnesses to take place.

Find them in: Deep fried foods, fast foods, commercially baked goods, and those prepared with partially hydrogenated oil, margarine and/or vegetable shortening. Note that items that list 0g trans fats on the label may still contain some amount of these toxic fats. This is because in the US, the government allows items containing less than 0.5g of trans fats to be declared as trans-fat free. Commercially prepared peanut butter is one good example. Your best bet is to read the ingredients list and make sure partially hydrogenated oil or vegetable shortening is not used.

Dairy Products

As much as 60% of the world's population cannot digest milk. In fact, researchers think that being able to digest milk beyond infancy is abnormal, rather than the other way round. Milk is also a common allergen that can trigger inflammatory responses, such as stomach distress, constipation, diarrhea, skin rashes, acne, hives and breathing difficulties in susceptible people.

Find them in: Milk and dairy products are as pervasive as foods containing partially hydrogenated oil or omega-3-deficient vegetable oil. Apart from obvious milk products like butter and cheese, foods with hidden dairy content include breads, cookies, crackers, cakes, cream sauces, and boxed cereals. Scanning the ingredients list is still the safest way to suss out milk.

Feedlot-Raised Meat

Commercially produced meats are feed with grains like soybeans and corn, a diet that is high in inflammatory omega-6 fatty acids but low in anti-inflammatory omega-3 fats. Due to the small and tight living environment, these animals also gain excess fat and end up with high saturated fats. Worse, to make them grow faster and prevent them from getting sick, they are also injected with hormones and fed with antibiotics. The result is one piece of meat which you and I should not be eating.

Find them in: Unless otherwise stated, most, if not all, beef, pork, and poultry you can find in the supermarkets and restaurants come from feedlot farms.

Red Meat & Processed Meat

Researchers at the University of California San Diego School of Medicine found that red meat contains a molecule that humans do not naturally produce called Neu5Gc. After ingesting this compound, the body develops anti-Neu5Gc antibodies – an immune response that may trigger chronic inflammatory response. Low-grade, simmering inflammation that will not go away has been linked to cancer and heart disease.

The link between processed meat consumption and cancer is even stronger. In the 2007 report by the World Cancer Research Fund and the American Institute for Cancer Research, processed meat has been stated as a convincing cause of cancers of the colon and rectum, and possibly of the esophagus and lungs too. Processed meat includes animal products that have been smoked, cured, salted, or chemically preserved.

Find them in: Common red meats are beef, lamb, and pork, while processed meats include ham, sausage and salami.

Alcohol

Regular high consumption of alcohol has been known to cause irritation and inflammation of the esophagus, larynx (voice box) and liver. Over time, the chronic inflammation promotes tumor growth and gives rise to cancer at the sites of repeated irritation.

Find them in: Beers, ciders, liquors, liqueurs, and wines.

Refined Grains

A lot of the grains we eat nowadays are refined. They are devoid of fiber and vitamin B compared to unpolished and unrefined grains that still have the bran, germ and the aleurone layer intact. This makes refined grains as good as refined sugars, which are practically empty calories. And like refined sugars, refined grains have a higher glycemic index than unprocessed grains and when they are consistently consumed, can hasten the onset of degenerative diseases like cancer, coronary disease, and diabetes.

Find them in: Products made from refined grains are almost everywhere. The common ones are: white rice, white flour, white bread, noodles, pasta, biscuits and pastries. To make things worse, many products with refined grains undergo further processing to enhance their taste and look, and are often loaded with excess sugar, salt, artificial flavors and/or partially hydrogenated oil in the process. A prime example is boxed cereals which contain substantial amounts of added sugar and flavorings.

Artificial Food Additives

Some artificial food additives like aspartame and monosodium glutamate (MSG) reportedly trigger inflammatory responses, especially in people who are already suffering from inflammatory conditions such as rheumatoid arthritis.

Find them in: Only packaged foods contain artificial food additives. If you need to buy them, read the labels carefully and weigh your risks. If you order Chinese takeaways, make sure you have the option to ask for no MSG. Otherwise, look elsewhere.

Glucose

https://www.naturalnews.com/2020-07-14-sugar-is-cancers-best-friend-research.html#
Sugar is cancer's best friend: Research reveals how it feeds tumors

(Natural News) We've known for quite some time that sugar essentially feeds cancer cells, with tumors preferring to use sugar fermentation as a source of energy. But now, studies are showing that it could, in fact, be the cause of the disease in the first place.

A study that was published in the Journal of Clinical Investigation illustrated how sugar could actually be the cause of cancer. They found that the activation of sugar-based metabolism within a cell, which is driven by the presence of higher quantities of glucose and an increase in glucose receptors on the surface of the cell membrane, can bring about cancer.

At the same time, the study revealed that interfering with the availability of sugar and its uptake into the cell can actually have the opposite effect, causing cancer cells to regress back to the way they were before cancer.

This research indicates that sugar is one of the main causes of the metabolic cell changes in the body that are consistent with the development of cancer. While that information is tremendously useful on its own, knowing that depriving cells of it could reverse cancer may be an even bigger game changer.

A different study that was published in the journal Science Signaling, meanwhile, built on earlier scientific literature showing that the cancer cells that multiply quickly tend to need a greater amount of sugar than normal cells. In the study, the researchers discovered that when cancer cells are deprived of sugar, it spurs a reaction across the cancer cell membrane that leads to the death of the cells.

Another study carried out by Belgian researchers over the course of nine years discovered that sugar stimulated cancer cells and caused them to multiply and expand rapidly.

Understanding the sugar-cancer connection could be a game-changer
A greater understanding of the connection between sugar and the onset and growth of cancer has the potential to dramatically change public health, especially in America, where people consume 160 pounds of the substance each year.

Unfortunately, sugar is highly addictive. In fact, some experts say that sugar could be as addictive as cocaine. That's because sugar releases dopamine and opioids in our bodies, activating the reward circuit that is a hallmark of addictive behavior.

In short, it gives you a type of high that you'll want to re-experience, so you repeat the behavior that gave you that feeling in the first place. Over time, you'll need to do it more and more to get the same effect, even as your body suffers from negative consequences such as headaches, weight gain, and all the other diseases excessive sugar consumption can lead to.

The American Heart Association recommends that women not eat more than six teaspoons of sugar per day; the limit for men is 9 teaspoons. The World Health Organization, meanwhile, recommends that everyone keep their daily intake of sugar at below 10 percent of their total energy intake.

Cancer is not the only reason to avoid sugar. Other negative health effects associated with the substance include a greater risk of obesity, type 2 diabetes, cardiovascular disease, quicker aging, and slower cognitive function.

Although it can sometimes feel like cancer is a disease that is beyond our control – and that may be true to an extent – scientists have found that lifestyle choices play a bigger role than genetics when it comes to our chances of developing cancer. Therefore, we have a lot more control than we think, and watching our sugar consumption is one of the best steps we can take if we want to prevent cancer.

Sources for this article include:

GreenMedInfo.com

NaturalNews.com

NaturalNews.com

Healthline.com

How I Killed the Cancer Stem Cells

This is what I do. Check with a Doctor to make sure it is safe. A lot of these are blood thinners

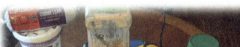
Things I buy at the grocery store

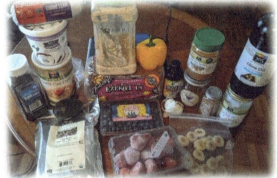

1) Garlic - **It passes through the <u>brain barrier</u> (BBB)** 1 or 2 cloves of <u>fresh garlic</u> a day. I have found out the hard way that it must be <u>fresh garlic</u>. It must be cut or smashed and let the garlic sit for about 15 minutes

2) Turmeric/Curcumin – I use 1-2 tablespoon of Turmeric. **Turmeric/Curcumin will cross the Brain Barrier (BBB)** I was confused. From the number of people asking me I think I should try and clear it up now. Turmeric does not fight cancer. A part of turmeric called curcumin is the cancer fighter. There is only 3%-5% of curcumin in turmeric. I do not take capsules I prefer Turmeric powder. Because I am indolent, I take 1-2 teaspoons of turmeric and a touch of black pepper is great for preventive measures or maintenance.
- If you have cancer, you need 8g-12g (8g = 3-2/3 teaspoons) of curcumin daily for 3 months *(that is all they tested it for and could not a*

problem: see GRAS in a later chapter) and a touch of black pepper to get it past the liver.

You cannot get there by taking Turmeric. It does not matter whether you are using turmeric powder, Turmeric Capsules, Golden Paste, or any other form. If you are fighting cancer the best way to do this is by taking **curcumin power.**

If you are not fighting cancer, then you need much less. Then you can use turmeric in capsules, Golden Paste, or whatever you use Turmeric in.

3) Ginger - (anti-inflammatory) I use 1-2 teaspoons of Ginger powder in my breakfast and 1-2 teaspoons in my smoothie.

4) Cayenne Pepper - (capsaicin) This is extremely hot. I use 1/8 of a teaspoon or I just sprinkle it in my breakfast.

5) Black Seed Oil *(Nigella sativa)* – I use 1 tablespoon of Black Seed Oil. It tastes horrible at first. I use it in a smoothie or with local honey.

6) Local Honey – ***Note: If you are a Diabetic or Pre-Diabetic you may not want to try Honey. You must check with a Doctor*** I use 1 tablespoon in a smoothie, 1 teaspoon in my oatmeal, 1 teaspoon on toast, 1 teaspoon in my coffee

7) Cinnamon – I use cinnamon in a smoothie, in my oatmeal, and on toast.

8) Avocado – I use 1 avocado a day. Usually at breakfast.

9) Blueberries – I use a hand-full of Blueberries in my oatmeal

10) Strawberries – I use a handful of frozen strawberries in a smoothie.

11) Coconut Oil - I use 1-2 tablespoons in a skillet for cooking

12) Olive Oil – I use 1-2 teaspoons in a skillet for cooking

13) Other - Almonds, Walnuts, Broccoli, Carrots, Dry Beans, Spinach, Sweet Potatoes, Pineapple, Beets, Oranges, Kale, Salmon, Swiss Chard – these are just a few.

Generally Recognized as Safe (GRAS)

https://www.fda.gov/food/food-ingredients-packaging/generally-recognized-safe-gras

"GRAS" is an acronym for the phrase Generally Recognized As Safe. Under sections 201(s) and 409 of the Federal Food, Drug, and Cosmetic Act (the Act), any substance that is intentionally added to food is a food additive, that is subject to premarket review and approval by FDA, unless the substance is generally recognized, among qualified experts, as having been adequately shown to be safe under the conditions of its intended use, or unless the use of the substance is otherwise excepted from the definition of a food additive.

- Under sections 201(s) and 409 of the Act, and FDA's implementing regulations in 21 CFR 170.3 and 21 CFR 170.30, the use of a food substance may be GRAS either through scientific procedures or, for a substance used in food before 1958, through experience based on common use in food Under 21 CFR 170.30(b), general recognition of safety through scientific procedures requires the same quantity and quality of scientific evidence as is required to obtain approval of the substance as a food additive. General recognition of safety through scientific procedures is based upon the application of generally available and accepted scientific data, information, or methods, which ordinarily are published, as well as the application of scientific principles, and may be corroborated by the application of unpublished scientific data, information, or methods.
- Under 21 CFR 170.30(c) and 170.3(f), general recognition of safety through experience based on common use in foods requires a substantial history of consumption for food use by a significant number of consumers.

Overview
- About the GRAS Notification Program
- How FDA's GRAS Notification Program Works
- FDA's Approach to the GRAS Provision: A History of Processes

GRAS Final Rule

- Federal Register Notice – the GRAS Final Rule (81 FR 54960 – August 17, 2016)
- Federal Register Notice - the GRAS Proposal (62 FR 18937 - April 17, 1997)
- Federal Register Notice - Substances Generally Recognized as Safe; Reopening of the Comment Period (75 FR 81536 - Dec 28, 2010)

Inventory for Human Food
- GRAS Notice Inventory

Regulatory and Policy Guidance
- Draft Guidance for Industry: Best Practices for Convening a GRAS Panel
- Regulatory Framework for Substances Intended for Use in Human Food or Animal Food on the Basis of the Generally Recognized as Safe (GRAS) Provision of the Federal Food, Drug, and Cosmetic Act
- Guidance for Industry: Frequently Asked Questions About GRAS for Substances Intended for Use in Human or Animal Food
- Guidance for Industry: Assessing the Effects of Significant Manufacturing Process Changes, Including Emerging Technologies, on the Safety and Regulatory Status of Food Ingredients and Food Contact Substances, Including Food Ingredients That Are Color Additives
- Guidance for Industry: Considerations Regarding Substances Added to Foods, Including Beverages and Dietary Supplements
- Draft Guidance for Industry: Providing Regulatory Submissions in Electronic or Paper Format to the Office of Food Additive Safety
    - See also: CFSAN Online Submission Module (COSM)
- Guidance for Industry: Frequently Asked Questions about FDA's Regulation of Infant Formula

Scientific Guidance
- Guidance for Industry: Recommendations for Submission of Chemical and Technological Data for Food Additive Petitions and GRAS Notices for Enzyme Preparations
- Guidance for Industry: Recommendations for Submission of Chemical and Technological Data for Direct Food Additive Petitions
- Guidance for Industry: Estimating Dietary Intake of Substances in Food
- Guidance for Industry: Summary Table of Recommended Toxicological Testing for Additives Used in Food

Regulations
- 21 CFR 181 - Prior Sanctioned Food Ingredients
- 21 CFR 182 - Substances GRAS in food

- 21 CFR 184 - Substances Affirmed as GRAS in Food
- 21 CFR 186 - Substances Affirmed as GRAS for Use in Food Packaging

Understanding FDA Food Labels

https://www.fda.gov/food/nutrition-education-resources-materials/new-nutrition-facts-label

From the Website listed above:

The U.S. Food and Drug Administration (FDA) has updated the Nutrition Facts label on packaged foods and drinks. FDA is requiring changes to the Nutrition Facts label based on updated scientific information, new nutrition research, and input from the public. This is the first major update to the label in over 20 years. The refreshed design and updated information will make it easier for you to make informed food choices that contribute to lifelong healthy eating habits.

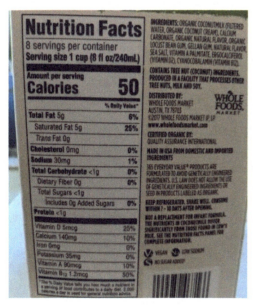

Learn about What's New with the Nutrition Facts Label, including details on calories, serving sizes, added sugars, and more.

Education Campaign

"The New Nutrition Facts Label: What's in it for You?" education campaign was developed by FDA to raise awareness about the changes to the Nutrition Facts label, increase its use, and help consumers, health care professionals, and educators learn how to use it as a tool for maintaining healthy dietary practices.

The education campaign includes outreach through many channels including social media, indoor/outdoor advertising, videos, and consumer-friendly downloadable educational materials.

In 2018, FDA announced the Nutrition Innovation Strategy, which sets a strategic course for taking action to reduce preventable death and disease related to poor nutrition. As part of the agency's strategy, this new campaign supports consumer education as a key element of FDA's ongoing public health efforts.

https://nutritionauthority.com/news/tips-for-understanding-the-nutrition-facts-labels/

From the Website listed above

The Nutrition Facts label packs in a great deal of information in a small area. It provides consumers with information about the foods that they consume. But is it as simple as it looks?

The nutrition label tells us the following:
- Serving size
- Calories
- Fat
- Cholesterol
- Sodium
- Carbohydrates
- Protein
- Vitamins and minerals

Fact or fiction

Food companies provide adequate information, but you always need to know how the information is packaged. At the top of each label, you will see Amount Per Serving. At first a food may seem low calorie in one serving, but a serving size sometimes is only ⅛ cup (C) How much is ⅛ C? Who eats ⅛ C? Will I feel full after eating ⅛ C, or will I need to eat several ⅛–1 C portions to satisfy my cravings? While the serving size is not the only dimension of choosing a product, it can skew how much you can or should eat in 1 day.

So how does this differ from portion size? Serving size is the amount of food that is determined by a food company in a standard measure, such as ¼ C, ⅓ C, ½ C, 2 tablespoons, etc. Portion size, on the other hand, is the amount of food that we choose to eat at one sitting.

Read before you eat but take the time to enjoy your food!

Fat and cholesterol

Fats are a mystery to some people. They taste so good, and many of us just cannot avoid them. But how much is too much, and what does each of the categories mean on the nutrition label?

Currently, the Nutrition Facts lists Total Fat, Saturated Fat, Trans Fat, and Cholesterol. Eating too much of these can increase your risk of **chronic diseases**, such as heart disease, some **cancers**, and high blood pressure.

While too much fat can have health consequences, we certainly need fats and cholesterol for our body to function properly, such as our hormones. In general, keep your % Daily Values (% DV) between 5%–20% for individual food items. Remember, if you eat more than one serving size, account for this in your calculations. If you have two serving sizes of 15% saturated fats/serving, then you are eating 30% of your % DV.

Dietary fiber, vitamins, and minerals

The first reason we read the nutrition label is to make right choices and to eat well. We should avoid or limit the consumption of certain foods, and we should eat more of other foods that contain **dietary fiber**, vitamins, and minerals. **Dietary fiber** often is found in carbohydrates, such as whole grains, fruits, and vegetables. The daily recommendation is 25 grams of fiber.

Many different vitamins are important, with vitamins A and C listed most often on the label. A deficiency of vitamin A, a fat-soluble vitamin, may cause night blindness and keratomalacia. A deficiency of vitamin C, a water-soluble vitamin, can cause scurvy.

Minerals also are included on labels, with calcium and iron listed most frequently. With the help of vitamins, minerals can boost the immune system, support growth and development, and help cells function normally. Calcium is very important for bone health, whether for building bone or for maintenance. Iron helps with hemoglobin, myoglobin, and enzymes, and lack of iron may result in anemia.

Helpful tips
Follow this helpful advice:

Eat a well-balanced diet
Limit fats in your diet to 5%–20% DV for individual food items
Aim to have 100% of the % DV of fiber, vitamins, and minerals in your diet—checking labels for the % DV in individual foods can help you achieve that goal

Read the label before you eat the food

The bottom line

The following chart of Percent Daily Values is based on a 2,000-calorie diet. It indicates how much a person should eat in fats, cholesterol, sodium, and carbohydrates.

Because the information is based on how much a person should eat on a 2,000-calorie diet, this footnote is always going to appear the same: *Percent Daily Values are based on a 2,000-calorie diet. Your Daily Values may be higher or lower depending on your calorie needs.

This information is helpful when you count how many grams or milligrams of each item you should consume. It also only helps if you consume a 2,000-calorie diet.

Recipes

This is what I do. Check with a Doctor to make sure it is safe. A lot of these are blood thinners. Note: If you are a Diabetic or Pre-Diabetic you do not want to do Honey

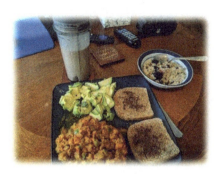

Cancer Stem Cells have recently been identified in several solid tumors, including: Brain, Breast, Colon, Ovary, Pancreas, Prostate, Melanoma, Multiple Myeloma, Non-melanoma skin cancer

James's Breakfast
In a skillet on low heat:
1 Tbs Coconut Oil
1 Tbs Extra Virgin Olive Oil
1 Tbs Avocado Oil
   Sausage – Plant-Based Ground or Regular Sausage
¼ Bell Pepper
1 Egg (Optional)
Tomatoes (Optional)

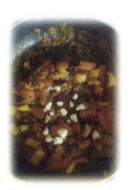

After it cooks for a while mix in:
1-2 Tbs Ginger
Splash Cayenne Pepper
1 tsp Curcumin
- If you are fighting cancer, use 4 tsp of Curcumin for 30 days

Splash of Black Pepper
Fresh Garlic (add it last to maintain its potency the less you cook it the better)
- Cut up the Garlic up let it sit for 15 minutes
- (I cut it up and let it sit before I start making breakfast)

James's Black Seed Oil Smoothie
1 cup unsweetened Coconut Milk
1 Tbs Honey
1 Tbs Black Seed Oil
1 Tbs Ginger
½ tsp Cinnamon
1 Banana
4-5 Strawberries
1-2 Tbs unsweetened Yogurt Alternative

James's Cinnamon Toast
1 Sprouted Grain Bread (Ezekiel)
1 tsp Honey
Almond Butter
Cinnamon

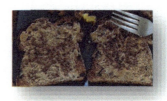

James's Oatmeal
1 ½ Cups Water
¼ Cup of Quick Cook Steel-Cut Oats
1 Tbs Honey
Dash Salt
Cinnamon
1 Scoop Blueberries

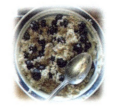

Turmeric Smoothie (Optional)
1 cup unsweetened Coconut Milk
1-2 Bananas
1 tsp Coconut Oil
1 tsp Honey
½ tsp Cinnamon
¼ clove of fresh Garlic
1/8 tsp Black Pepper
1 tsp Ginger
1-2 tsp Turmeric

If you are fighting cancer you need to substitute 8-12 grams (about 4 teaspoons) of Curcumin a day for 3 months

The rest of the day I try to stay on an ant-inflammation diet (with some cheating):
Grapes, Carrots, Salmon, Halibut, Sweet Potatoes, Broccoli, Brussel Sprouts, Beets,

Salads, Olives, Tuna Salad, Chicken Salad, Dips with Carrots Slices, Almonds, Walnuts, Dry Beans, Spinach, Oranges, Kale....Anything Anti-Inflammatory

The Gift That Will not Stop Giving: Chemotherapy and Radiation

It is bad enough I suffer from "Chemo Brain", but I never expected the results from radiation. With chemotherapy I suffer from Short Term Memory Loss, I leave words out when I type, I have to put my finger on each word when I read, My Math skills aren't what it once was. I figured out how to get around these things. Thank God for Smart Phones

I had all my teeth before I got cancer. I think I have had 11 extractions since 2014. My Dentist said it is due the radiation that I received back in 2013. She says it can go on forever. I have another tooth that is going to be extracted sometime in the future.

I complained to my Oncologist because I was hoarse all the time. She sent me to an Ear, Nose, and Throat Specialist. As it turns out one of my vocal cords is partially paralyzed. It never ends. ***Please do not do Chemotherapy and Radiation***.

Apoptosis

Remember this definition you will see it a lot in the next few pages:

The definition of ***Apoptosis***:
: a genetically directed process of cell self-destruction that is marked by the fragmentation of nuclear DNA, is activated either by the presence of a stimulus or removal of suppressing agent or stimulus, is a normal physiological prosses eliminating DNA-damaged, superfluous, or unwanted cells, and when halted (as by gene mutation) may result in uncontrolled cell growth and tumor formation

--also called cell suicide, programmed cell death DPG

My Treatment Plan

My Oncologist sent me to Neurological Surgeon for second opinion on if I should resume Chemotherapy. I refused twice even though he said I might die. Here are the Doctor's visits. Now he is a believer.

2016/01/11
Mr. McCraw is a 57-year-old male who presents for evaluation of a left frontal Glioblastoma Multiforme. I think his current imaging supports tumor progression

2016/03/14
Mr. McCraw is a 57-year-old male who presents for follow-up of a left frontal Glioblastoma Multiforme. I continue to think his current imaging supports tumor progression.
I discussed the situation with him. He is not very interested in intervention at this point. He understands the ramifications of this, which include death. I will see him in two months with repeat imaging. He will call in the interim with any questions or concerns. All discharge instructions were given, and all questions were answered. He is to visit the West Clinic tomorrow.

2016/05/23

Mr. McCraw is a 57-year-old male who presents for follow-up of a left frontal Glioblastoma Multiforme. His imaging shows improvement.

Once again, I discussed the situation with him. He is not very interested in intervention at this point. He understands the ramifications of this, which include death. I will see him in two months with repeat imaging. He will call in the interim with any questions or concerns. He will continue to see Dr. _____, as instructed. All discharge instructions were given, and all questions were answered. He is to visit the West Clinic tomorrow.

2016/08/29

Mr. McCraw is a 57-year-old male who presents for follow-up of a left frontal Glioblastoma Multiforme. His imaging shows improvement.

I will see him in three months with repeat imaging. He will call in the interim with any questions or concerns. He will continue to see Dr. _____, as instructed. All discharge instructions were given, and all questions were answered. He is to visit the West Clinic tomorrow.

2017/11/06

Mr. McCraw is a 58-year-old male who presents for follow-up of a left frontal Glioblastoma Multiforme. His imaging shows improvement.

I will see him in three months with repeat imaging. He will call in the interim with any questions or concerns. He will continue to see Dr. _____ as instructed. All discharge instructions were given, and all questions were answered. He is to visit the West Clinic tomorrow.

2018/05/07

Mr. McCraw is a 59-year-old male who presents for follow-up of a left frontal Glioblastoma Multiforme. His imaging shows improvement.

I will see him in six months with repeat imaging. He will call in the interim with any questions or concerns. He will continue to see Dr. _____ as instructed. All discharge instructions were given, and all questions were answered.

2018/11/05

Mr. McCraw is a 59-year-old male who presents for follow-up of a left frontal Glioblastoma Multiforme. His imaging is satisfactory.

I will see him in six months with repeat imaging. He will call in the interim with any questions or concerns. He will continue to see Dr. _____ as instructed. All discharge instructions were given, and all questions were answered.

2019/05/01

Mr. McCraw is a 60-year-old male who presents for follow-up of a left frontal Glioblastoma Multiforme. His imaging is satisfactory.

I will see him in six months with repeat imaging. He will call in the interim with any questions or concerns. He will continue to see Dr. _____ as instructed. All discharge instructions were given, and all questions were answered.

2020/07/22

Mr. McCraw is a 61-year-old male who presents for follow-up of a left frontal Glioblastoma Multiforme. I will see him in October with repeat imaging

2020/10/21

Mr. McCraw is a 61-year-old male who presents for follow-up of a left frontal Glioblastoma Multiforme. His imaging is satisfactory. I will see him in six months with repeat imaging.

2021/04/19

Mr. McCraw is a 62-year-old male who presents for follow-up of a left Frontal Glioblastoma Multiforme. His imaging is satisfactory. I will see him in one year with repeat imaging.

There Is No Cure For Cancer

Cancer is a chronic metabolic disease. Chronic diseases can be controlled, not cured. There is no cure for cancer

First, according to Doctor Aggarwal PhD, Doctor David Servan-Schreiber, Morgan Freeman - Actor, Bill Henderson, Doctor Richard Beliveau, Doctor Michael Roizen M.D., Doctor Oz, Johns Hopkins University, **there is no cure for cancer**. Everyone has cancer cells. You cannot cure something that everyone has. Doctor Bharat B. Aggarwal, PhD says that if you control your inflammation, you control cancer. I believe this. Everyone is looking for a cure for cancer. They are running marathons, researching, and wishing for cure. They might find something to fight the symptoms, but I think finding a cure would be like finding a cure for the common cold.

Every person has cancer cells in their body. There cancer cells do not show up in the standard test until they have multiplied to a few billion.

Cancer cells occur between 6 to more than 10 times in a person's lifetime.

When the person's immune system is strong the cancer cells will be destroyed and prevented from multiplying and forming tumors.

Glioblastoma Multiforme

A Glioblastoma Multiforme Grade 4 tumor. That was the cancer that I have. When I first went to the hospital and was diagnosed with a brain tumor. My surgeon decided he wanted to wait until after he did the surgery. He could have drilled a hole in my skull and found out. He decided that he would have to do surgery anyway. I had a craniotomy: a surgical operation of the skull. I found out my prognosis through my Oncologist after the surgery. I decided right then that I was going to beat it. I was diagnosed July 22, 2013. My prognosis was 14 months. My surgery was on October 13, 2013. It has been quite the adventure. The only symptom I had were seizures.

https://www.ncbi.nlm.nih.gov/pmc/articles/PMC4497660/

From the website above:

A very small proportion of patients diagnosed with glioblastoma (GBM) survive more than 3 years. Isocitrate dehydrogenase 1 or 2 (IDH1/2) mutations define a small subgroup of GBM patients with favorable prognosis. However, it remains controversial whether long-term survivors (LTS) are found among those IDH1/2 mutated patients.

Results
Seventeen patients with survival >3 years were identified (8.2% of the total series). The median overall survival in long-term survivors was 4.6 years. Subgroup analysis found that the median age at diagnosis was significantly higher for non long-term survivors (non-LTS) compared to LTS (60 versus 51 years, $p <0.03$). The difference in the rate of IDH mutation between non-LTS and LTS was statistically not significant (1.16% versus 5.9%, $p = 0.144$). Among LTS, 10 out of 16 tumors presented a methylation of MGMT promoter.
Conclusions
This study confirms that long-term survival in GBM patients is if at all only weakly correlated to IDH-mutation.

Glioblastoma
Medical Condition

A cancerous tumor which develops in the brain.

Very rare (Fewer than 20,000 cases per year in US)

Requires lab test or imaging

Treatments can help manage condition, no known cure

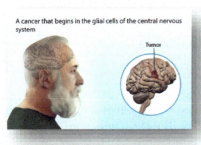

A cancer that begins in the glial cells of the central nervous system

Can last several years or be lifelong

The exact cause is not known. It is associated with certain genetic changes, and environmental factors. Characterized by headache, nausea, dizziness, blurred vision, and seizures. Treatment includes medications such as surgery, chemotherapy, and radiation.

Symptoms
- Persistent headaches
- Nausea
- Vomiting
- Blurred vision
- Changes in cognitive abilities
- Memory loss
- Personality changes
- Seizures
- Muscle weakness
- Difficulty in speaking

Treatments

Treatment is difficult due to the fact that the tumor cells are very resistant to conventional therapies. Further, many drugs cannot cross blood-brain barrier to act on the tumor.

Medication
- Chemotherapy: To kill cancerous cells. Temozolomide

Medical procedures: Neurosurgery

Therapies: Radiation therapy

Causes
The exact cause of this condition is unknown
- It is associated with genetic disorders such as neurofibromatosis, tuberous sclerosis, and Li- Fraumeni syndrome
- Previous radiation therapy increases risk
- It is more common in males
- Exposure to smoking, pesticides or working in a petroleum refining increases risk
- Associated with viruses such as cytomegalovirus, SV40
- More common in Caucasian and Asian ethnicities

https://cancerwall.com/glioblastoma-multiforme-life-expectancy-stage-4-survival-rate-symptoms-prognosis/

This is from the above website
Stage 4 glioblastoma multiforme Life expectancy
Stage 4 glioblastoma multiforme is the last stage of brain tumor. For the patient in IV stage of glioblastoma multiforme, the rate of survival diminishes. With treatment, the patient can hardly live two years as the disease is not curable. In this stage, the tumor travels, and spreads in another part of the body. In generally the life expectancy of the patient detected with stage for cancer varies from few months to two years. The average life expectancy of the patient above 60 years is one years. If an adult detected with the diseases is of 40 years of age, then chances are there that he can survive up to five more years.

Prognosis and Survival Rate
Once the disease is diagnosed then the patient can survive 3 months without any treatment. But with the treatment and medical consultation, the patient suffering from glioblastoma multiforme can survive up to 1-2 years. Increased intracranial pressure and cerebral edema increases the death rate. The brain tumors which are caused due to glioblastoma multiforme are generally malignant in nature and grow aggressively. Young patients suffering from the condition have high chances of survival whereas older patents do not have a favorable outcome. Infants born with glioblastoma multiforme have only 30 percent survival rate and with treatment they can survive for five more years. The survival chances in glioblastoma multiforme generally depend on the stage and condition of the disease.

Ludwig Center

https://med.stanford.edu/ludwigcenter/overview/theory.html
The Stem Cell Theory of Cancer
Once again this is my favorite analogy from the Ludwig Center it says it all: "An analogy would be a weeding technique that is evaluated based on how low it can chop the weed stalks—but no matter how low the weeds are cut, if the roots aren't taken out, the weeds will just grow back"

Research has shown that cancer cells are not all the same. Within a malignant tumor or among the circulating cancerous cells of a leukemia, there can be a variety of types of cells. The stem cell theory of cancer proposes that among all cancerous cells, a few acts as stem cells that reproduce themselves and sustain the cancer, much like normal stem cells normally renew and sustain our organs and tissues. In this view, cancer cells that are not stem cells can cause problems, but they cannot sustain an attack on our bodies over the long term.

The idea that cancer is primarily driven by a smaller population of stem cells has important implications. For instance, many new anti-cancer therapies are evaluated based on their ability to shrink tumors, but if the therapies are not killing the cancer stem cells, the tumor will soon grow back (often with a vexing resistance to the previously used therapy).

Another important implication is that it is the cancer stem cells that give rise to metastases (when cancer travels from one part of the body to another) and can also act as a reservoir of cancer cells that may cause a relapse after surgery, radiation or chemotherapy has eliminated all observable signs of a cancer.

One component of the cancer stem cell theory concerns how cancers arise. In order for a cell to become cancerous, it must undergo a significant number of essential changes in the DNA sequences that regulate the cell. Conventional cancer theory is that any cell in the body can undergo these changes and become a cancerous outlaw. But researchers at the Ludwig Center observe that our normal stem cells are the only cells that reproduce themselves and are therefore around long enough to accumulate all the necessary changes to produce cancer. The theory, therefore, is that cancer stem cells arise out of normal stem cells or the precursor cells that normal stem cells produce. Thus, another important implication of the cancer stem cell theory is that cancer stem cells are closely related to normal stem cells and will share many of the behaviors and features of those normal stem cells. The other cancer cells produced by cancer stem cells should follow many of the rules observed by daughter cells in normal tissues. Some researchers say that cancerous cells are like a caricature of normal cells: they display many of the same features as normal tissues, but in a distorted way. If this is true, then we can use what we know about normal stem cells to identify and attack cancer stem cells and the malignant cells they produce.

Backup

Garlic

I switched from fresh garlic to an unscented garlic supplement. The cancer came back. The good news is that I realized that it was the garlic and not the standard treatment of chemo and radiation.

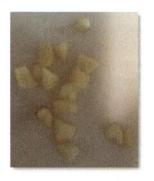

Cut and peel the **clove** of garlic and let it sit for 15 minutes before consuming. This time allows for the release of an enzyme (allinase) that produces the anti-cancer compounds. You can eat it raw, cook with it, make a smoothie with garlic. I would not try cooking it awfully long, especially on a high heat. The less you cook garlic the better.

It passes through the brain barrier (BBB), and it actually attacks the cancer cells including the **cancer stem cells**. Allicin (from garlic) induces caspase-mediated *apoptosis* in cancer cells

I did nothing but Garlic from December 2013 through December 2015. Garlic Supplements will **not** work.

Turmeric/Curcumin

I was confused and from the number of people asking me. I think I should try and clear it up now. **Turmeric** does **not** fight cancer. It would be like taking a couple of aspirin and expecting it to beat cancer. A part of **turmeric** called **curcumin** is the cancer fighter. There is only 3%-5% of curcumin in turmeric. It would be impossible to take that much Turmeric. I was taking **Turmeric** when supposed to be taking **Curcumin.** I equate that to the fact that it was the other things I did to fight cancer. I started doing Garlic the right way. I also added Ginger and Cayenne Pepper. I do not take capsules I prefer Turmeric powder. Because I am cancer free (indolent) I take 1-2 tablespoons of turmeric and a touch of black pepper is great for preventive measures or maintenance.

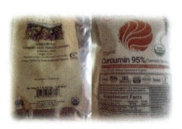

I buy Turmeric and Curcumin at Amazon

- If you have cancer, you need 8g-12g (8g = 3-2/3 teaspoons) of curcumin daily for 3 months (that is all they tested it for and could not a problem: see GRAS in a later chapter) and a touch of black pepper to get it past the liver. You cannot get there by taking Turmeric. It does not matter whether you are taking turmeric, Turmeric Capsules, Golden Paste, or any other form. If you are fighting cancer the best way to do this is by taking curcumin power.

If you are not fighting cancer. Then you need much less. Then you can use turmeric in capsules, Golden Paste, or whatever

Turmeric/Curcumin will cross the Brain Barrier (BBB) you will have to add black pepper to get it past the liver. You can use Coconut Oil or Olive Oil. It actually attacks the cancer cells including the cancer stem cells. Curcumin kills tumor cells by modulating several cells signaling pathways such as it inhibits activation of NF-$\varkappa$B leading to *apoptosis* in the tumor cells. Further, curcumin induces apoptosis through the release of cytochrome c and inhibits Akt in renal cancer cells

Turmeric/Curcumin has been fighting cancer since **1815**. There is no money in it. So, the FDA does not get the attention. So is Not FDA approved

https://www.thehindu.com/sci-tech/health/medicine-and-research/curcumin-a-wonder-drug-in-waiting/article7719513.ece

This is from the above website:
The fact remains that curcumin is not an approved drug even for a single ailment, although **USFDA** has classified it as a **GRAS (Generally Regarded As Safe)** molecule. Data is available from over 100 clinical trials (completed and ongoing), including **cancers** and other diseases, using curcumin alone or in combination with existing therapy. The data indicate positive trends, but with the invariable conclusion that larger clinical trials with appropriate randomized designs are needed.

This is the stage we have reached and remained after decades of research; **curcumin was discovered in 1815!** A molecule that is beneficial for a variety of ailments, based on a science that cannot explain its diverse drug targets, an action that defies pharmacological parameters and above all a drug that is **cheap** and **not easily patentable** as such, will never make the grade in the eyes of multinational pharmaceutical companies.

But what is preventing Indian drug companies from looking at curcumin as an approved drug for specific ailments in the clinic? It is here that there is an opportunity for the Indian Council of Medical Research (ICMR) to step in and take steps to promote curcumin as a unique molecule to treat specific diseases.

The best option appears to conduct clinical trials with curcumin as an adjunct therapy with the existing drugs. It can work synergistically as an anti-inflammatory molecule and can decrease the toxicity and resistance to the primary drug. It can be a unique antidote to treat and prevent drug resistance. This will be a great contribution which India can make to the cause of affordable therapy with justifiable pride in the wisdom of ancient Indian medicine.

US patent office withdraws patent on Indian herb
K. S. Jayaraman
Nature volume 389, page6(1997) Cite this article

NEW DELHI

India has forced the US Patent and Trademark Office (PTO) to revoke a contentious patent it granted two years ago to researchers in the United States on the use of powdered turmeric (Curcuma longa) for wound healing.

The PTO withdrew the patent on 13 August after a year-long legal battle with India's Council of Scientific and Industrial Research (CSIR), which argued that turmeric, a native Indian plant, had been used for centuries by its people for wound healing, and so lacked the "novelty" criterion required for patenting.

The Indian agency hired a US patent lawyer and spent $15,000 to fight the case, which it supported with documents ranging from scientific publications to books on home remedies and ancient Ayurvedic texts on Indian systems of medicine.

Indian scientists claim this is the first time that a move in the United States to patent a traditional remedy from the developing world has been successfully overturned. Earlier efforts by an international coalition of environmentalists to get the US patents on products of the neem tree cancelled ended in failure (Nature 377, 95; 95; 1995).

The CSIR's director, Ragunath Mashelkar, said the success of the case had far-reaching consequences for the protection of the traditional knowledge base, "not only in India but in other Third World countries". He said the case also highlights the importance of documenting traditional knowledge, to provide evidence of prior knowledge.

The turmeric patent was granted in 1995 to two researchers, Soman K. Das and Harihar Kohli of the University of Mississippi Medical Center. Their six patent claims covered the oral and topical use of turmeric powder to heal surgical wounds and ulcers. Das and Kohli contested CSIR's objections, but the patent office rejected all their claims.

The patenting of traditional remedies from developing countries became a global issue after patents were granted for neem. These patents were upheld because they covered novel processes for increasing the useful life of azadirachtin, neem's active ingredient.

Mashelkar says that India fought the turmeric patent not for financial reasons, but to uphold "national pride" and to dispel unfounded fears that India was incapable of protecting its traditional knowledge base.

In cooperation with other agencies, the CSIR has already launched a program to analyze 490 medicinal plants and place the information on CD-ROM. This will be made available to European and US patent offices as a reference guide.

Ginger

Ginger kills **cancer stem cells** and prevents them from building up resistance to cancer treatment. Evidence suggest that ginger and its active constituents suppress the growth and induce *apoptosis* of variety of **cancer types including skin, ovarian, colon, breast, cervical, oral, renal, prostate, gastric, pancreatic, liver, and brain cancer.**

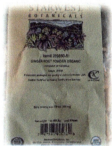

This is the Ginger I use. I buy it Amazon

https://en.wikipedia.org/wiki/Gingerol
The following is from the above website

Gingerol
Phytochemical Compound

Gingerol, properly as-gingerol, is a phenol phytochemical compound found in fresh ginger that activates spice receptors on the tongue. Molecularly, gingerol is a relative of capsaicin and piperine, the compounds which are alkaloids, though the bioactive pathways are unconnected. It is normally found as a pungent yellow oil in the ginger rhizome but can also form a low-melting crystalline solid. This chemical compound is found in all members of the Zingiberaceae family plant and is high in concentrations in the grains of paradise as well as an African Ginger species.

In a pre-clinical meta-analysis of gingerol compounds anticancer, anti-inflammatory, anti-fungal, antioxidant, neuroprotective and gastroprotective properties were reported, which include studies in-vitro and in-vivo. A few in-vivo studies have proposed that gingerols facilitate healthy glucose regulation for diabetics. Many studies have been around the effects of gingerols on a wide range of cancers including leukemia, prostate, breast, skin, ovarian, lung, pancreatic and colorectal. There has not been much clinical testing to observe gingerols physiological impacts in humans.

While many of the chemical mechanisms associated with the effects of gingerols on cells have been thoroughly studied, few have been in a clinical setting. This is due to the high variability in natural phytochemicals and the lack of efficacy in research. Most herbal medicine, which include gingerols, are under the restrictions of the Food and Drug Administration in the United States and experimental methods have not held up to scrutiny which has decreased the value in phytochemical research. Herbal medicine is untested for quality assurance, potency, and effectiveness in clinical settings due to a lack of funding in eastern medical research. Most research on [6]-Gingerol has been on either mouse subjects (in-vivo) or on cultured human tissue (in-vitro) and may be used in the future to discuss possible applications for multi-target disease control.

An investigation scrutinizing gingerol's anti-fungal capabilities remarked that an African species of ginger tested higher in both gingerol and shogaol compounds than the more commonly cultivated Indonesian relative. When tested for the anti-fungal properties the African ginger combated against 13 human pathogens and was three times more effective than the commercial Indonesian counterpart. It is thought that gingerol compounds work in tandem with the other phytochemicals present including shogaols, paradols and zingerone.

A few established cellular pathways effected by [6]-gingerol that result in apoptosis of a cancerous cell. ABBREVIATIONS: CDK: Cyclin-dependent kinase; PI3K: Phosphoinositide 3-kinase; Akt: Protein kinase B; mTOR: Mammalian target of rapamycin; AMPK: 5'adenosine monophosphate-activated protein kinase; Bax: Bcl-2-associated X protein; Bcl-2: B-cell lymphoma 2.

In a meta-analysis looking at many different phytochemical effects on prostate cancer, two specific studies using mice observed [6]-gingerol compounds induced apoptosis in cancer cells by interfering with the mitochondrial membrane.[13] There were also observed mechanisms associated with the disruption of G1 phase proteins to stop the reproduction of cancer cells which is also an associated benefit of other relevant anticancer studies. The main mechanism by which gingerol phytochemicals act on cancer cells seems to be protein disruption. The anti-carcinogenic activity of [6]-gingerol and [6]-paradol was analyzed in a study observing the cellular mechanisms associated with mouse skin cancer which targeted the activator proteins associated with tumor initiation. Gingerol compounds inhibited the transformation of normal cells into cancer cells by blocking AP-1 proteins and when cancer did develop paradol encouraged apoptosis due to its cytotoxic activity. [6]-Gingerol exhibits cell cycle arrest capabilities, apoptotic action and enzyme-coupled cell signaling receptor degradation in cancer cells. Gingerol has been observed to stop proliferation through inhibiting the translation of Cyclin proteins necessary for replication during G1 and G2 phase of cell division. To promote apoptosis in cancer cells Cytochrome C is ejected from the mitochondria which ceases ATP production leaving a dysfunctional mitochondria. The Cytochrome C assembles an apoptosome which activates the Caspase-9 and initiates an executioner Caspase cascade, effectively breaking down DNA into histones and promoting apoptosis. [6]-Gingerol also inhibits the anti-apoptotic Bcl-2 proteins on the surface of mitochondria, which in turn increases the capabilities for the pro-apoptotic Bcl-2 proteins to initiate cell death. Cancer cells exhibit high amounts of growth hormone activator proteins that are expressed through enzyme-coupled signaling pathways. By halting the phosphorylation of PI-3-Kinase the Akt protein cannot bind with its PH domain, effectively deactivating the downstream signal. Successively keeping Bad proteins bound to anti-apoptotic proteins which keeps them from promoting cell growth, consequently, a double negative cellular signaling pathway to promote apoptosis.

Cayenne Pepper

It is an anti-inflammatory. It was found that it disrupted mitochondrial function and induced **apoptosis** (programmed cell death). Cayenne Pepper contains **Capsaicin**. It can **cross the Blood Brain Barrier (BBB)**. Cayenne pepper increases blood flow. Cayenne Pepper is one of the oldest and most powerful healing remedies in the world.

Capsaicin demonstrates the ability to inhibit the growth of cancer cells; research suggests that the compound promotes *apoptosis* – the death of cancer cells. In 2010 researchers from the UCLA School of Medicine studied breast cancer cells and found that capsaicin not only retarded their growth and arrested their ability to travel, but also increased the degree of apoptosis. The results of this research were published in the January 2010 issue of the journal "Oncogene."

Black Seed Oil

(Nigella sativa) Thymoquinone is the active main constituent in black seed oil. It is an anti-inflammatory. I believe it improved my memory.

Black seed oil causes *apoptosis*, so it promotes a systematic elimination of cells which are no longer needed, are old, or unhealthy (as cancer cells), and does not release toxins into the body. Moreover, this beneficial oil is also responsible for the control of the Akt pathway, that it, the process that helps the survival of normal and cancer cells.

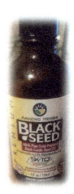

https://www.nootropedia.com/black-seed-oil/
An excerpt from the website above:
In an October 2016 study, authors recognized that black seed oil (and specifically the psychoactive compound thymoquinone) could cross the blood brain barrier effectively and protect against brain damage, reduce oxidative stress... The same study goes on to say that black seed oil can have an anti-tumor (anti-cancer) effect when studied in animal models.

Finally, black seed oil benefits include boosts for cognition and general learning ability. One study showed that 20 weeks of consistent black seed supplementation could improve memory formation [7]. Another study in humans showed a 13.5 – 14.7% boost in memory tests

https://worldhealth.net/news/using-black-seed-oil-treat-cancer/
An excerpt from the website listed above:
Thymoquinone has been shown to modulate nine out of the ten hallmarks of cancer. Experts are urging more research into thymoquinone, which is the active main constituent in black seed oil, for adjuvants to pharmaceutical cancer treatments, and signaling pathways that black cumin seed oils play in being a cancer killer.

Cancer depending on what form of cancer, in the most basic explanation is cells gone wrong, the cause of is most often not discovered of which malignant cancers are the ones to be most worried about.

Many studies have shown the effects of Nigella sativa on various different cancer cells, and the list is long offering up over 57 reviewed papers on the subject finding black cumin to be effective against cancers such as blood, breast, colon, pancreatic, lung, leukemia, skin, fibrosarcoma, renal, prostate, and cervical cancer.

Anticancer effects are mediated through different modes of action including cell cycle arrest, apoptosis induction, ROS generation and anti-metastasis/anti-angiogenesis, and anti-proliferation. Additionally, anticancer activity was also found to exhibited through modulation of multiple molecular targets including p53, p73, PTEN, STAT3, PPAR, activation of caspases, and generation of ROS.

Extracted from Nigella sativa thymoquinone has been investigated for its antioxidant, anti-inflammatory, and anticancer properties since the 1960 in vitro and vivo models as it may act as a superoxide and free radical scavenger to go along with preserving activity of various antioxidant enzymes such as glutathione-S-transferase, glutathione peroxidase, and catalase. Its anti-inflammatory and antioxidants effects have been reported in various disease models of diabetes, carcinogenesis, asthma, and encephalomyelitis.

In a large review of studies conducted on black cumin investigating its role as an anticancer agent it was explained that many active ingredients have been found within the seeds containing fixed and essential oils, proteins, alkaloids and saponin which described quantification of 4 pharmacologically important components: thymoquinone, dithymoquinone, thymohydroquinone, and thymol within the oil of the black seed oil by HPLC.

Black cumin has been shown to be provide effective protection against the toxicity of the drug cyclophosphamide, suggesting administration of NSO of TQ can lower CTX induced toxicity by upregulation of antioxidant mechanisms, indicating potential to minimize toxic effects of treatment with anticancer drugs.

Nigella sativa oil has been recommended as a natural radioprotective agent against immunosuppressive and oxidative effects of ionizing radiation.

Nigella sativa has been shown to inhibit colon carcinogenesis of rats in postinitiation stage in epilepsy studies, that may be associated with suppression of cell proliferation in the colonic mucosa with no adverse side effects.

Antineoplastic activities of thymoquinone have been demonstrated in multiple cancers, including cancer cells have been shown to be unable to produce fibroblast growth factor and protein collagenase after being incubated with Nigella extract.

Angiogenesis was blocked by thymoquinone in vitro and vivo preventing angiogenesis in xenograft human prostate cancer mouse models, and inhibited human prostate tumor growth at low doses with almost no chemotoxic side effects.

Thymoquinone has also been shown to suppress growth and invasion, and to induce apoptosis of glial tumors cells via degrading tubulins and inhibiting 20S proteasome, telomerase, autophagy, FAK and metalloproteinases.

Thymoquinone was shown to increase sub-G1 accumulation and annexin-V positive staining indicating apoptotic induction. TQ was observed to be more potent than cisplatin in elimination of SiHa cells via apoptosis with down regulation of Bcl-2 proteins.

Thymoquinone triggers apoptotic cell death in human colorectal cancer cells via p53-dependent mechanisms, indicating TQ is an antineoplastic and pro-apoptotic against colon cancer cell line HCT116. Effects are modulated by Bcl-2 proteins linked to p53, supporting using TQ for the treatment of colon cancer, meaning that black seed oil kills cancer cells.

Autophagy is inhibited by thymoquinone, and it induces cathepsin mediated caspase independent cell death in glioblastoma cells.

Black seed oil has much potential in regarding to healing to cancers. So much data and research are available that it makes one wonder why cancer patients are not routinely being treated with black cumin seed oil.

Materials provided by:
Note: Content may be edited for style and length.

https://www.naturalnewsblogs.com/why-arent-hospitals-treating-cancer-with-black-seed-oil/

https://www.detoxnaturalliving.com/blackseedoilmasterguide.html

Local / Organic Honey
- Note: If you are a Diabetic or Pre-Diabetic you may not want to try Honey. You must check with a Doctor
Natural products such as honey have potential anticancer effect.

Honey is composed of various sugars, flavonoids, phenolic acids, enzymes, amino acids, proteins, and miscellaneous compounds. Its composition varies according to floral sources and origin. It has been shown to have anti-inflammatory, antimicrobial, antimutagenic, antioxidant, and antitumor effects. The phenolic contents of honey have been reported to have antileukemic activity against different types of leukemic cell lines. Its anticancer activity has been proved against various cancer cell lines and tissues, such as breasts, colorectal, renal, prostate, endometrial, cervical, and oral cancer

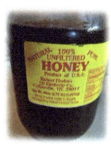

DISCLAIMER: People that are diabetic should talk to their Doctor before they do Honey. I just want to let you know.

Believe it or not, Local Honey is good for fighting cancer. You better be sure it is pure Local Honey or Organic Honey and not just the "store bought" honey that has been pasteurized or has antibiotics. It is best if you know the beekeeper or someone that knows he has a good reputation. Local Honey or Organic Honey is a safe bet. There are certain rules they must follow to get the USDA to approve the honey. According to **Anya Vien** "Your honey can be tainted with lead and antibiotics. Spiking honey is a common practice in the US. It means that corn syrup or other sweeteners have been added to honey to make it more affordable. Most honey sold in America is not exactly what the bees produce." According to **Dr. Heather Paulson**, ND, FABNO is a board- certified naturopathic oncologist "Yes! A lot of honey on the shelf is being adulterated with fructose syrup and high fructose syrup. It may be best to buy your honey directly from a local beekeeper. Plus, supporting local beekeepers supports local hives."

I use 1 teaspoon of honey as a sweetener in my coffee, I use 1 teaspoon in my oatmeal, 2 teaspoons on toast with cinnamon and Almond Butter and 1 tablespoon of honey in a smoothie. According to **Dr Ron Fessenden, MD, MPM** "Generally, three to five tablespoons of honey a day is sufficient. A good regimen to follow is to consume a tablespoon or two of honey in the morning with fruit or yogurt or cereal. Another tablespoon should be consumed at bedtime"

https://www.ncbi.nlm.nih.gov/pmc/articles/PMC3065157/
Recently, Tarek et al. showed that honey could induce *apoptosis* inT24, RT4, 253J, and MBT-2 bladder cancer cell lines. They showed significant inhibition of the proliferation of T24 and MBT-2 cell lines by 1%—25% honey and of RT4 and 253J cell lines by 6%—25% honey.

https://spoonuniversity.com/lifestyle/raw-honey-vs-organic-honey-wtf-is-the-difference#:~:text=Honey%20that%20is%20labeled%20as%20organic%20according%20to,chemicals%20or%20located%20far%20away%20from%20any%20present.

Raw Honey vs Organic Honey: WTF is the Difference?
What's all the buzz about?

Jennie Toutoulis
Fairfield University

"Organic Honey: Honey that is labeled as **organic** according to the USDA was made from a bee farm that follows the organic livestock standards. These standards state that the hives must be free of chemicals or located far away from any present. Also, the flowers that the bees will be getting nectar from cannot be sprayed with chemicals and the bees cannot be given antibiotics.
The Problem
While raw and organic honey have their own guidelines to make them different from each other, there is a problem: the label. There are no strict legal requirements for labeling honey as raw or organic. Honey can be labeled as being raw or organic without these strict requirements because bee farmers understand the beneficial process of making both types and follow them anyway."

"So, when it comes to your grocery shopping, raw or organic honey are both great choices compared to the thinner honey that has been pasteurized"

"Finally, all the buzz about raw honey vs organic honey has come to an end. While very similar, there are some minor differences that separate raw from organic honey. But since there aren't any legal guidelines distinguishing the two, both are pretty sweet additions to your grocery cart"

https://anyavien.com/a-lit-of-honey-brands-with-no-pollen/#:~:text=Honey%20has%20a%20dirty%20little%20secret%3A%20Your%20honey,added%20to%20honey%20to%20make%20it%20more%20affordable.

According to Anya Vien
Disclaimer: The information on This Website (anyavien.com) has not been evaluated by the FDA. The information on This Website is not intended to diagnose, treat, cure, or prevent any disease. The information on This Website is not medical

advice, nor is it a substitute for medical advice or for consultation with a qualified physician; if you have medical concerns or symptoms, or are considering use of herbs or supplements, please seek advice from a qualified physician. This Website makes no actual recommendations or claims whatsoever as to the use of herbs, nor makes any guarantees whatsoever as to either the efficacy of such products nor as to the accuracy of any claims made about them. This Website and its contents are provided for general information, reportage, background research and entertainment purposes only. This Website's owner specifically disclaims responsibility for any consequences of using This Website and its contents.

"Your honey can be tainted with lead and antibiotics. Spiking honey is a common practice in the US. It means that corn syrup or other sweeteners have been added to honey to make it more affordable. Most honey sold in America is not exactly what the bees produce"

"Honey and cancer have a sustainable inverse relationship. Carcinogenesis is a multistep process and has multifactorial causes. Among these are low immune status, chronic infection, ***chronic inflammation***, chronic non healing ulcers, obesity, and so forth. There is now sizeable evidence that honey is a natural immune booster, natural ***anti-inflammatory*** agent, natural antimicrobial agent, natural cancer "vaccine," and natural promoter for healing chronic ulcers and wounds. Though honey has substances of which the most predominant is a mixture of sugars, which itself is thought to be carcinogenic, it is understandable that its beneficial effect as anticancer agent raises skeptics. The positive scientific evidence for anticancer properties of honey is growing. The mechanism on how honey has anticancer effect is an area of great interest. Among the mechanisms suggested are inhibition of cell proliferation, induction of ***apoptosis***, and cell-cycle arrest. Honey and cancer have sustainable inverse relationship in the setting of developing nations where resources for cancer prevention and treatment are limited"

https://drheatherpaulson.com/honey-cancer-shocking-truth/#:~:text=%20A%20study%20published%20in%20the%20journal%20Evidence-Based,Cause%20cancer%20cell%20death%20through%20apoptosis%20More%20

Doctor Heather Paulson says:
Does it need to be a special type of honey?

Studies have looked at Manuka honey, Bush Honey, and natural honey. All seem to be effective against cancer cells and in improving immune status. However, the darker the honey, the more positive plant chemicals it had. So, look for darker honey.

What's in Honey that helps it protect us against cancer?

Some of the polyphenols (aka plant chemicals) that have been studied in honey are:
- Caffeine acid: a powerful antioxidant
- Chrysin: can also reduce aromatase enzyme hormone production
- Caffeic Acid Phenyl Esters (CAPE): has been studied against glioblastoma
- Quercetin: effective in cell cultures against many cell lines including pancreatic cancer, prostate cancer, breast cancer, colon cancer, and skin cancer.
- Apigenin: studied again many cancer types.

Is there anything I should watch out for when it comes to honey?

Yes! A lot of honey on the shelf is being adulterated with fructose syrup and high fructose syrup. It may be best to buy your honey directly from a local beekeeper. Plus, supporting local beekeepers supports local hives.

Bees need our help to stay alive! They are facing their own health epidemic right now.

About the Author: Dr. Heather Paulson

Dr. Heather Paulson, ND, FABNO is a board-certified naturopathic oncologist and an expert in combining natural therapies, nutrition, exercise, and emotional healing. She creates a strategy for dealing with cancer just for YOU. In her 10 years of clinic experience, she's helped thousands of people with cancer. She has dedicated her life and medical training helping those moving through the cancer experience.

Cinnamon

Cinnamon has various biological functions including antioxidant, anti-microbial, anti-inflammation, anti-diabetic and anti-tumor activity.

https://www.ncbi.nlm.nih.gov/pmc/articles/PMC2920880/

From the website listed above:

Background

Cinnamomum cassia bark is the outer skin of an evergreen tall tree belonging to the family Lauraceae containing several active components such as essential oils (cinnamic aldehyde and cinnamyl aldehyde), tannin, mucus, and carbohydrate. They have various biological functions including antioxidant, anti-microbial, anti-inflammation, anti-diabetic and anti-tumor activity. Previously, we have reported that anti-cancer effect of cinnamon extracts is associated with modulation of angiogenesis and effector function of CD8+ T cells. In this study, we further identified that anti-tumor effect of cinnamon extracts is also link with enhanced *pro-apoptotic* activity by inhibiting the activities NFκB and AP1 in mouse melanoma model.

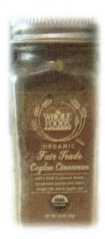

Cinnamon extract strongly inhibited tumor cell proliferation in vitro and induced active cell death of tumor cells by up-regulating ***pro-apoptotic*** molecules while inhibiting NFκB and AP1 activity and their target genes such as Bcl-2, BcL-xL and surviving. Oral administration of cinnamon extract in melanoma transplantation model significantly inhibited tumor growth with the same mechanism of action observed in vitro.

Conclusion

Our study suggests that anti-tumor effect of cinnamon extracts is directly linked with enhanced ***pro-apoptotic*** activity and inhibition of NFκB and AP1 activities and their target genes in vitro and in vivo mouse melanoma model. Hence, further elucidation of active components of cinnamon extract could lead to development of potent anti-tumor agent or complementary and alternative medicine for the treatment of diverse cancers.

Cinnamomum cassia bark is the outer skin of an evergreen tall tree belonging to the family Lauraceae. Its extracts contain several active components such as essential oils (cinnamic aldehyde and cinnamyl aldehyde), tannin, mucus, and carbohydrates [5,6]. They have various biological functions including antioxidant, anti-microbial, anti-inflammation, anti-diabetic effects, and anti-tumor activity. However, for the development of cinnamon as CAMs for cancer treatment, further studies are necessary such as elucidation of working mechanisms and characterization of active compounds directly linked with anti-tumor activity.

Cancers are the most life-threatening health problems in the world. There have been many trials to treat cancers through modulation of anti-tumor immune response, apoptosis, and anti-tumor proteins. Tumor cells are generally resistant to ***apoptosis***; hence selective killing of tumor cells by promoting ***apoptosis*** pathway is an attractive and effective way for development of anti-cancer agents. NFκB and AP1 constitutively active in many kinds of cancers and play critical roles in tumor development and progression through modulation of their target genes involved in angiogenesis, metastasis, and cell survival [19-21].

Recently we have reported that anti-cancer effect of cinnamon extracts is associated with modulation of angiogenesis and effector function of CD8+ T cells [22]. In this study we further identified that anti-tumor effect of cinnamon extracts is also linked with their enhanced ***pro-apoptotic*** activity by inhibiting the activities of NFκB and AP1 in mouse melanoma model.

Avocado

Molecules derived from avocados have been found to target the stem cells of acute myeloid leukemia (AML), according to a study published in the journal Cancer Research on Monday. The lipid found in avocado joins just a handful of drug treatments available that attack leukemia stem cells directly while leaving healthy cells unharmed.

https://blog.cirm.ca.gov/2015/06/18/holy-guacamole-nutrient-in-avocado-kills-cancer-stem-cells/

An excerpt from the website listed above:

As if the news couldn't get any better, research published this week now suggests that a nutrient found in avocado can kill <u>cancer stem cells</u> – a cell type thought to be the source of a **cancer's unlimited growth and spread**

The study, reported in Cancer Research by a Canadian research team at the University of Waterloo, focuses on a particularly deadly form of blood cancer called acute myeloid leukemia (AML). Often striking adults over 65, AML has a poor prognosis with only 10% survival after five years for this age group.

The cancer is caused by rapid, abnormal growth of white blood cells in the bone marrow that eventually crowds out normal blood cells leading to a deterioration of vital functions of the blood like carrying oxygen to the body. Chemotherapy or bone marrow transplants are standard treatments but unfortunately, even when successful, a majority of AML patients will relapse.

Though they make up a tiny portion of the leukemia, **cancer stem cells** are thought to be the main culprits behind AML relapse due to their stem cell-like ability for unlimited growth. The research team identified a nutrient in avocados called avocatin B with the ability to kill AML **cancer stem cells**. The killing mechanism of avocatin B was pinpointed to its disruption of the mitochondria, the cell's energy "factory", in leukemia cells, which led to cell death. As senior author Professor Paul Spagnuolo points out in a university press release, this cancer killing property of avocatin B promises to have limited side effects:

https://www.curejoy.com/content/avocado-seed-benefits/

We haven't found any mention of avocado seeds for cancer in folk medicine literature, but a 2013 study found that ethanol extracts of the avocado fruit and seed could induce death (*apoptosis*) in cells affected by leukemia or blood cancer. The researchers even suggest using avocado as an alternative treatment for leukemia.

Blueberries

https://csn.cancer.org/node/297330
From the above website:
Blueberries Kill Cancer Cells and Reduce Tumor Size

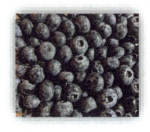

Numerous studies have shown that at least one third of cancers would be linked to the kinds of food that we habitually eat. According to the World Cancer Research Fund International, our diet plays an important role in developing certain cancers. Data even show that a diet rich in fruits and vegetables divides the risk in half; that's more effective than any conventional prevention method.

You may ask why blueberry is among the top anticancer foods. Many plants contain molecules that can not only prevent the development of cancerous cells but also slow their progression in individuals who already have the disease. Among twenty fruits, blueberry is ranked first for its powerful antioxidant capacity. Closely follow cranberry, blackberry, raspberry, and strawberry.

Although research on the anticancer properties of blueberry is in its infancy, some scientific studies suggest that anthocyanidins (pigments found in certain plant which have amazing health benefits) contained in blueberries also have an important anti-cancer potential which patients and healthy people can greatly benefit from. The anticancer potential of the berries is also explained by its anti-inflammatory action.

Anthocyanidins, as well as other molecules present in blueberry, would slow the progression of cancer by blocking the development of blood vessels feeding the malignant cells. This antiangiogenic process deprives cancer cells of their supply of oxygen and nutrient molecules needed to reproduce, which makes it a powerful anticancer food.

Blueberries are amongst the most consumed berries not only in the United States but also in many other parts of the world. They are rich in phenolic compounds, thus high in antioxidants. According to a review published by the Department of Nutrition, Food and Exercise Sciences, from The Florida State University, on Pubmed, "evidence from in vitro, in vivo and a few clinical studies suggest that blueberries and their active constituents show promise as effective anti-cancer agents, both in the form of functional foods and as nutritional supplements."

Although more studies are needed, this mini study shows the carcinogenesis of blueberries works by inhibiting the production of pro-inflammatory molecules, which is the genesis of the formation of all malignant tumors. The berries also help stop oxidative stress, DNA damage, and cancer cell proliferation, while at the same time increase the natural programmed cell death (*apoptosis*) which cancerous cells defect. When consider defective *apoptosis* is the backbone of the occurrence and proliferation of malignant tumors, the work of blueberries in re-establishing it should be greatly considered.

Another study was conducted by the Department of Biochemistry (U38-FCT), Faculty of Medicine of the University of Porto, Portugal, to investigate the anticancer properties of an anthocyanin-pyruvic acid adduct extract from blueberry in fighting certain types of cancer such as breast cancer. At the end, the scientists conclude the following:

"An anthocyanin extract from blueberry (extract I) and an anthocyanin-pyruvic acid adduct extract (extract II) were tested on two breast cancer cell lines (MDA-MB-231 and MCF7). Proliferation was assessed by SRB assay and ^{3}H-thymidine incorporation. Caspase-3 activity was determined in the presence of both extracts. In both cell lines, extracts I and II significantly reduced cell proliferation at 250 μg/mL, after 24 h of cell incubation. Caspase-3 activity was not altered by the extracts (250 μg/mL) in either cell line, with the exception of extract II in MCF-7, which increased its activity... Both extracts (250 μg/mL) demonstrated significant antiinvasive potential in both cell lines."

In other studies, it is observed in laboratory that regular consumption of fresh blueberry juice, raspberry and cranberry would slow the growth of human cancer cells mainly in the stomach, prostate, and colon (bowel). Leukemic cells also reduced.

It is clear eating blueberries regularly may not only helps prevent formation of cancer in healthy individuals but also stop or reduce the proliferation of the cancerous cells patients who are already struggling with the condition.

https://www.ncbi.nlm.nih.gov/pmc/articles/PMC5103680/
Excerpts from above websites:
Effects of blueberries on migration, invasion, proliferation, the cell cycle, and **apoptosis** in hepatocellular carcinoma cells

Strawberries

Helped prevent early lesions from developing into tumors.

https://www.ncbi.nlm.nih.gov/pmc/articles/PMC3468438/

Previous studies suggest that consumption of berry fruits can have beneficial effects against diseases such as cancer. Berries contain multiple phenolic compounds, which contribute to their biological properties. It has been suggested that bioactive components of berry invoke anti-cancer effects through various complementary and overlapping mechanisms of action including the induction of metabolizing enzymes, modulation of gene 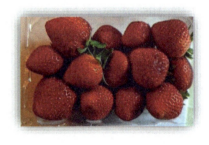 expression etc. However, their definitive mechanism of action is largely unknown.

Strawberries are a good source of natural antioxidants, which can be linked to the level of phenolic compounds in these fruits. A recent study showed that strawberry extracts exhibit a higher level of antioxidant capacity against free radical species including superoxide radicals, hydrogen peroxide, hydroxyl radicals, and singlet oxygen. Strawberries contain antioxidants, such as vitamin C, hydroxycinnamic acids, anthocyanins and flavonoids. Besides, due to relatively high content of ellagic acid, an antioxidant that can exert antimutagenic and anticarcinogenic effect, it has been a preferred target for cancer studies. A study has also shown that strawberries have potent anti-proliferative activity on human liver cancer cells, HepG2. However, there are no studies to investigate its anticancer potential and the mechanism by which it exerts its effect.

Various phytochemicals and chemically synthesized small molecules induce *apoptosis*, largely through the activation of intrinsic pathway. Intrinsic apoptotic pathway involves a variety of stimuli from inside the cells like DNA damage, ROS generation etc. The major players of this pathway include BCL2 family of proteins, which are mainly classified as proapoptotic and antiapoptotic proteins, based on their activity. An imbalance in the ratio between these classes of proteins leads to damage of mitochondrial membrane integrity resulting in CYTOCHROME C release and CASPASE 9 followed by CASPASE 3 activation [20].

In the present study, we show that extracts prepared from Indian strawberry fruits induce cytotoxicity by activating intrinsic pathway of *apoptosis*, through a p53 independent mechanism in breast cancer cells. MESB also interferes with progression of tumors in breast cancer mouse models and results in the extended lifespan without affecting other cellular functions and body weight. Most importantly, we also provide evidence that strawberry consumption can delay tumorigenesis in mice.

Coconut Oil

The Journal Cancer Research has found an active anti-cancer component in coconut oil. Lauric acid, a major ingredient of this oil, has been shown in a University of Adelaide study to kill over 90% of the colon cancer cells after just two days of treatment.

https://coconutoil.com/study-coconut-oil-improves-memory-and-brain-function/

This was an in-vitro (lab culture) study titled "Coconut oil protects cortical neurons from amyloid beta toxicity by enhancing signaling of cell survival pathways" and also published recently (2017).

From their observations of adding coconut oil to cultures with rat brain neurons they observed:

Coconut oil and its medium chain fatty acids (MCFAs) protect against amyloid beta (Aβ) induced neurotoxicity in primary rat cortical neurons.
Amyloid beta is a protein fragment precursor to amyloid plaque and brain tangles that manifest dementia. Coconut oil also stimulated Akt protein enzyme pathways,

which play a key role in multiple cellular processes such as glucose metabolism, *apoptosis*, cell proliferation, transcription, and cell migration.

The researchers also observed coconut oil's medium chain fatty acids (MCFAs) or medium chain triglycerides (MCTs) ketone body influence as energy for a brain that is glucose impaired by insulin resistance, considered brain diabetes or type 3 diabetes.

Olive Oil

Oleocanthal is a polyphenol found in extra-virgin olive oil. 1 It has gained notoriety in the wellness community for its antimicrobial, antioxidant, anti-inflammatory, anticancer and neuroprotective effects

https://www.ncbi.nlm.nih.gov/pmc/articles/PMC2677148/

Olive oil intake has been shown to induce significant levels of *apoptosis* in various cancer cells. These anti-cancer properties are thought to be mediated by phenolic compounds present in olive. These beneficial health effects of olive have been attributed, at least in part, to the presence of oleuropein and hydroxytyrosol. In this study, oleuropein and hydroxytyrosol, major phenolic compound of olive oil, was studied for its effects on growth in MCF-7 human breast cancer cells using assays for proliferation (MTT assay), cell viability (Guava ViaCount assay), cell *apoptosis*, cellcycle (flow cytometry). Oleuropein or hydroxytyrosol decreased cell viability, inhibited cell proliferation, and induced cell *apoptosis* in MCF-7 cells. Result of MTT assay showed that 200 μg/mL of oleuropein or 50 μg/mL of hydroxytyrosol remarkably reduced cell viability of MCF-7 cells. Oleuropein or hydroxytyrosol decrease of the number of MCF-7 cells by inhibiting the rate of cell proliferation and inducing cell apoptosis. Also, hydroxytyrosol and oleuropein exhibited statistically significant block of G1 to S phase transition manifested by the increase of cell number in G0/G1 phase.

Oatmeal

Is good for digestion, Energy, Weight loss, Blood sugar and diabetes, Blood pressure, and **Cancer**

I Do not buy the instant oats. I use organic Steel-cut oats. I use cinnamon and blueberries or blackberries local or organic honey.

https://www.livestrong.com/article/555498-does-oatmeal-fight-cancer

According to Serena Styles and the Harvard School of Public Health

"Antioxidants, such as those found in oatmeal, might help fight cancer, as well as several other diseases according to the **Harvard School of Public Health**. Antioxidants neutralize toxins in your body that increase the risk of cancer, known as free radicals. These free radicals can damage your DNA cells, which may lead to cancer. According to the National Cancer Institute, antioxidants help block damage done by free radicals, fighting cancer, and reducing its risk. One of the best ways to include antioxidants in your diet is eating foods rich in them, as studies show antioxidant supplements might be harmful. Oats contain a higher level of antioxidants than most other grains, making oatmeal an ideal choice"

Coffee

There is a big question over coffee being carcinogenic. I must admit if it were not for coffee, I couldn't make it of bed. I keep it to 1-2 cups of coffee a day. Researchers have been investigating the links between coffee and cancer for decades. But there is still a lot they do not know. In 2016, an expert panel convened by the International Agency for Research on Cancer (IARC) – the arm of the World Health Organization that is responsible for assessing whether certain substances cause cancer – could not conclude that drinking coffee is carcinogenic based on the current evidence available. See more in Back-up Reference section.

https://www.cancer.org/latest-news/coffee-and-cancer-what-the-research-really-shows.html

Coffee and Cancer: What the Research Really Shows
Apr 3, 2018

Researchers have been investigating the links between coffee and cancer for decades. But there is still a lot they don't know. In 2016, an expert panel convened by the International Agency for Research on Cancer (IARC) – the arm of the World

Health Organization that is responsible for assessing whether certain substances cause cancer – could not conclude that drinking coffee is carcinogenic based on the current evidence available.

And now the coffee-cancer connection is in the news again. A California court ruling last week about a coffee warning related to a chemical formed during the roasting process (called acrylamide) has raised questions among consumers.

So, what do coffee drinkers need to know? In this interview, American Cancer Society researchers, **Susan Gapstur, PhD, and Marjorie McCullough, ScD**, provide insights into what studies to date really show when it comes to coffee and cancer, and discuss what another research is still needed.

Q. What does the research show about the link between coffee and cancer?

A. Numerous studies have shown that coffee drinking is associated with a lower risk of dying from all causes of death. However, associations with cancer overall or with specific types of cancer are unclear. In 2016, an expert working group convened for the International Agency for Research on Cancer Monographs Programme reviewed the world's body of human and laboratory research on coffee drinking and cancer risk, and they found the evidence of carcinogenicity of coffee drinking to be **"unclassifiable"**.

They also found that **coffee drinking is not a cause of female breast, pancreas, and prostate cancers**, but may reduce the risk of uterine endometrium and liver cancers. The evidence was judged to be inadequate for other cancer types. Reasons for the lack of convincing evidence included inconsistent results across studies and issues with data quality.

Additionally, because smokers also tend to be coffee drinkers, it is difficult to completely account for tobacco use in studies of coffee and strongly tobacco-related cancers. These issues can be addressed by examining risk in non-smokers, or with detailed statistical adjustment for smoking. For example, early research suggested that coffee increased the risk of bladder cancer, but the true causal factor was later found to be smoking.

Q. And, what about research into whether coffee is associated with a lower cancer risk?

A. Recent studies find that coffee may lower the risk of several types of cancer, including **head and neck, colorectal, breast, and liver cancer**, although the potential beneficial effects of coffee are not completely understood. Hundreds of biologically active compounds including caffeine, flavonoids, lignans, and other polyphenols are found in roasted coffee. These and other coffee compounds have been shown to increase energy expenditure, inhibit cellular damage, regulate genes involved in DNA repair, have **anti-inflammatory** properties, and/or inhibit **metastasis**, among other activities. There is also evidence that coffee consumption is associated with lower risk of insulin resistance and type 2 diabetes, which have been linked to higher risks of colorectal, liver, breast, and endometrial cancer incidence and/or mortality.

Q. What is acrylamide and what do we know about its link to cancer?

A. Coffee can contain acrylamide, a chemical that is also used in certain industrial processes and has been commercially available since the 1950s. In addition to coffee, acrylamide is also found in French fries (frying causes acrylamide formation), toasted bread, snack foods, like potato chips and pretzels, crackers, biscuits, cookies, and cereals, and in tobacco products. Acrylamide is classified by IARC as a "probable carcinogen," based primarily on genotoxicity experiments in animals. In 2002, Swedish scientists discovered that acrylamide could be formed from asparagine (an amino acid) and sugar during high-heat cooking. This discovery led to intensified research into the association between acrylamide intake from diet and cancer risk in humans. In 2011 and 2014, two large studies summarized the evidence in humans and found no association between dietary acrylamide and risk of several cancers.

Q. What is the bottom line when it comes to coffee – should people be worried about drinking it?

A. Overall, it seems that there may be health benefits to coffee drinking, but the risks remain unclear. Further research is needed to more fully understand the biologic mechanisms underlying associations of coffee drinking, acrylamide exposure, and cancer risk. Regardless, when considering behavioral approaches to reduce cancer risk, it is worth keeping in mind that preventing smoking initiation and improving smoking cessation rates remain the most important ways to reduce cancer mortality rates worldwide. After smoking, we also know that certain healthy lifestyle habits can significantly minimize cancer risk: these include limiting alcohol consumption, maintaining a healthy body weight throughout adulthood, being physically active, and consuming a mostly plant-based diet. If you are concerned about acrylamide exposure, you may also consider limiting intake of French fries, chips, and cookies, which is consistent with the American Cancer Society's dietary guidelines.

Red Meat

In the U.S.A we eat far too much meat. It is in our breakfast, lunch, dinner, snacks. Red Meat is okay only if it is minimally processed, hormone free and antibiotic free. There is a catch. When the FDA labels meat claiming the meat is hormone free. That could mean that no extra hormones given. The USDA allows some products to be labeled "Raised without Hormones" "Raised without Antibiotics" The animals were grown without antibiotics that are used for animal health or treatment of diseases. It is important to understand the labeling.

Most fast foods, restaurants, grocery stores do not meet these requirements. The bottom line is to check labels and eat far less meat. I eat some meat but keep it to a minimum. I found a veggie sausage (not the frozen kind) that I use in my breakfast. It looks and tastes like regular sausage.

Avoid These at All Costs
Processed Foods and Meats, Fast Foods

https://www.healthline.com/nutrition/grass-fed-vs-grain-fed-beef#grassfed-vs-grainfed

The difference between grass- and grain-fed cattle

In the United States, most cows start living similar lives.

The calves are born in the early spring, drink milk from their mothers, and are then allowed to roam free and eat grass or other edible plants they find in their environment.

This continues for about 7–9 months. After that, most conventionally raised cows are moved to **feedlots**.

Large **feedlots** are called concentrated animal feeding operations (CAFOs). There, the cows are kept in **confined stalls, often with limited space**.

They are rapidly fattened with grain-based feeds that are usually made from a base of soy or corn. Typically, their diet is also supplemented with small amounts of dried grass.

The cows live in these **feedlots** for a few months before being brought to a slaughterhouse.

Of course, it's not that simple. The different feeding practices are complicated and varied.

For example, grass-fed beef in Australia may not be directly comparable to US products, and grass-fed beef isn't necessarily pasture-raised. Not all grass-fed cows can graze outdoors.

In fact, the term grass-fed isn't clearly defined.

That said, grass-fed cows eat (mostly) grass, while grain-fed cows eat (mostly) an unnatural diet based on corn and soy during the latter part of their lives.

To maximize growth, the cows are often given drugs, such as antibiotics and growth hormones.

As of January 1st, 2017, the Food and Drug Administration (FDA) passed new legislation known as the Veterinary Feed Directive.

According to this legislation, antibiotics that are considered important in human medicine need to be administered under the oversight of a licensed veterinarian and cannot be used for growth promotion).

SUMMARY Most cows start on a pasture, drinking milk and eating grass. However, conventionally raised cows are later moved to **feedlots** and fed mainly grain-based feeds.

Bread

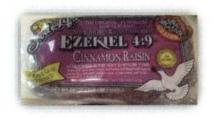

I use Ezekiel Bread most of the time. It has no sugar. You must keep it in your refrigerator. It is made from freshly sprouted live grains and contains no flour. There are times when I use "Nature's Own" for breads, hot-dog buns and hamburger buns. It needs to have a minimum amount of sugar. 0 grams of sugar is preferred.

https://www.eatthis.com/bread-store-bought/

18 Best and Worst Store-Bought Breads, According to Experts

TIFFANY GAGNON

When most people embark on a new diet, the first thing that seems to get the boot is the bread. But carbs shouldn't always be the dietary scapegoat. Dropping them from your diet will depress your taste buds, and it could prevent you from achieving lasting, healthy weight loss. Instead of cutting carbs completely, simply switch to one of the healthiest bread loaves you can buy in the bread aisle.

How nutritionists choose the healthiest bread.
Not all loaves of bread are created equal, and what makes the healthiest bread lies in the ingredients. "Bread has a bad rap for being full of fillers and additives, high in carbs, and sometimes even sugar. When grocery shopping, it is important to keep your eyes out for ingredients such as partially hydrogenated oils, high fructose corn syrup, and soy—I never buy bread that has those ingredients on the label!" says registered dietitian Kelly Springer, MS, RD, CDN.

Certain slices will offer your body absolutely no nutrition while others can fill you up with fiber and energy-boosting whole grains. (Yes, there are best bread loaves for weight loss out there!) Not to mention, some varieties today go even further and pack healthy, satiating fats into the mix by adding nuts and seeds.

So, if you absolutely can't live without bread, use this list of 8 healthiest bread options you can find at the grocery store, and 10 you should avoid at all costs.

The 8 Healthiest Breads You Can Buy At the Store

1. Best Low Sodium: Ezekiel 4:9 Low Sodium Sprouted Whole Grain Bread
Ezekiel 4:9 Low Sodium Sprouted Whole Grain - best bread
NUTRITION PER 1 SLICE: 80 calories, 0.5 g fat, 0 g sat fat, 0 mg sodium, 15 g carbs, 3 g fiber, 0 g sugar, 4 g protein

2. Best Sprouted Grain: Ezekiel 4:9 Sesame Sprouted Whole Grain Bread
Ezekiel 4:9 Sesame Sprouted Whole Grain - best bread
NUTRITION PER 1 SLICE: 80 calories, 0.5 g fat, 0 g sat fat, 80 mg sodium, 14 g carbs, 3 g fiber, 0 g sugar, 4 g protein

3. Best Whole Wheat: Arnold Whole Grains 100% Whole Wheat Bread
Arnold Whole Grains 100% Whole Wheat - best bread
NUTRITION PER 1 SLICE: 110 calories, 1.5 g fat, 0 g sat fat, 180 mg sodium, 20 g carbs, 3 g fiber, 3 g sugar, 5 g protein

4. Best Whole Grain: Nature's Harvest Stone Ground 100% Whole Wheat Bread
Nature's Harvest Stone Ground 100% Whole Wheat - best bread
NUTRITION PER 2 SLICES: 140 calories, 2 g fat, 0 g sat fat, 200 mg sodium, 29 g carbs, 4 g fiber, 5 g sugar, 7 g protein

5. Best Seeded: Eureka! Seeds The Day, Organic
Eureka! Seeds The Day bread - best bread
NUTRITION PER 1 SLICE, 18 OZ PACKAGE: 80 calories, 2 g fat, 0 g sat fat, 120 mg sodium, 13 g carbs, 2 g fiber, 3 g sugar, 4 g protein

6. Best High-Fiber Bread: Nature's Own Double Fiber Wheat
Nature's Own Double Fiber Wheat - best bread
NUTRITION PER 1 SLICE: 50 calories, 0.5 g fat, 0 g sat fat, 120 mg sodium, 11 g carbs, 4 g fiber, 0.5 g sugar, 3 g protein

7. Best Multigrain: Shiloh Farms Sprouted 7 Grain Bread, Organic
Shiloh Farms Sprouted 7 Grain - best bread
NUTRITION PER 1 SLICE: 100 calories, 0 g fat, 0 g sat fat, 120 mg sodium, 18 g carbs, 3 g fiber, <1 g sugar, 6 g protein

8. Best High-Protein Bread: Arnold Whole Grain Double Protein
Arnold Whole Grain Double Protein - best bread
NUTRITION PER 1 SLICE: 100 calories, 1.5 g fat, 0 g sat fat, 150 mg sodium, 18 g carbs, 3 g fiber, 2 g sugar, 7 g protein

Gluten

https://www.oncologynutrition.org/erfc/healthy-nutrition-now/foods/does-gluten-cause-cancer

There is no connection between gluten and risk of most cancers. The exception is intestinal cancer, and even then, gluten only increases risk if a person has celiac disease, or true gluten intolerance.

In fact, numerous observational studies show that the more whole grains a person eats, including the gluten-containing grains (wheat, rye, barley, and triticale), the lower his or her risk of most cancers. This is true for some of the most common types of cancer, such as breast, prostate, and colon cancers, as well as for less common cancers, such as cancer of the pancreas. Whole grains contain fiber, which can stabilize blood sugar and hormone levels.

Whole grains and fiber help us stay full, making it easier to maintain a healthy body weight. And whole grains contain hundreds of nutrients that appear to prevent damage in the body that can lead to cancer and its progression. For all these reasons, whole grains—those with gluten and without—should be part of a healthy diet.

There is one situation in which gluten must be avoided completely: celiac disease, or true gluten intolerance. In this situation, exposure to gluten can lead to a host of health problems, including increased risk of intestinal cancer. However, even in people with celiac disease, gluten is not associated with increased risk of most other cancers.

But for people with celiac disease, gluten must be avoided to limit the risk of other devastating health effects, such as malnutrition, anemia, osteoporosis, neurological effects, alopecia (hair loss), skin rashes, and thyroid problems.

As a final note, well over half of all people following a gluten-free diet do not have celiac disease. This means people may be needlessly avoiding healthy foods that are linked with lower risk of many chronic diseases, including cancer. If you suspect you have gluten-intolerance, talk to your doctor. A blood test can help diagnose the condition. If you do not have celiac disease, but gluten-containing grains do not agree with you, try cutting back. You may not need to eliminate them completely. If you still find these foods cause you problems, make an appointment with a registered dietitian.

A registered dietitian can help you sort out your digestive issues, and design a healthy, cancer-risk reduction diet that helps you feel your best.
Submitted by Suzanne Dixon, MPH, MS, RD, on behalf of the ON

Keto Diet

https://www.organicauthority.com/energetic-health/3-reasons-the-ketogenic-diet-might-be-the-ultimate-anti-inflammatory-cancer-fighting-protocol

This is from the website listed above:

1. It's anti-inflammatory, and cancer is an inflammatory disease.
Some of the biggest proven benefits of the keto diet are linked to general inflammation, a problem stemming in part from increased stress and poor diet that plagues many living in America today.
One 2015 study from the National Institutes of Health linked the ketogenic diet to the release of the ketone beta-hydroxybutyrate (BHB), which can block the NLRP3 inflammasome, an immune system receptor that's linked to inflammation.
"In summary, by encouraging ketosis, we can discourage the number of NLRP3 flares in the body," explains Dr. Laurie Steelsmith, author of Growing Younger Every Day: The Three Essentials Steps for Creating Youthful Hormone Balance At Any Age.
She notes that evidence in favor of keto's anti-inflammatory benefits only continues to grow. It's thus no surprise that the keto diet might be beneficial for cancer, seeing as cancer is, in fact, an inflammatory disease.
The National Cancer Institute writes that chronic inflammation can cause DNA damage and lead to cancer, and several academic papers, including a 2002 article in the journal Nature delve into this connection.
To stave off cancer, then, whether before or after diagnosis, an anti-inflammatory protocol like the ketogenic diet is key.

Zupec-Kania notes that while she hasn't had the opportunity to work with people attempting to use healthy diets such as the keto diet to prevent illness, she has seen the healing effects of keto on patients who have already been diagnosed with cancer first-hand.

"The main thing that we report, at least initially is that they just have much more energy," she says. She also shares that she has worked with several patients who have seen other benefits to transitioning to keto, including a woman with stage-four metastatic liver cancer who has already undergone two trials of chemotherapy.

"She's elderly, and she's doing beautifully," says Zupec-Kania. "I've been working with her for several months now, and one would think that if the cancer were getting worse, she wouldn't be doing so well."

"Probably the most outstanding case that is documented is a woman who contacted me, she has a rare breast cancer, and found out that chemo for this type of cancer is not that beneficial," Zupec-Kania continues. "She asked the doctor to give her some time doing thyrotherapy, which is where you freeze the tumors, and then keto diet, which is where I came in. She's six, seven years out."

When practiced properly, the keto diet's anti-inflammatory benefits may be promising, then, in both preventing and accompanying diagnosed patients on their journey to restored health.

2. The ketogenic diet works best with whole foods, and whole foods help fight cancer.

Most experts agree that some of the "keto" recipes that people post on the Internet are far from the ideal ketogenic diet.

"I've seen some really bad ketogenic diets that I don't think are anti-inflammatory," says Zupec-Kania. "I think the poor aspect of their diet probably cancels out the potential benefits of ketosis."

"I try to say to people, do you have any idea how much medicine you're putting into your body every day? We call it food, but it's medicine."

In some cases, she explains, this medicine is good, as in the case of vitamin-rich keto-friendly grass-fed animal fats, fruits, and vegetables. In some cases, however, it's like succumbing to the adverse side effects of a drug: a recent study found that the consumption of ultra-processed foods led to a 12 percent increase in risk of developing cancer.

"I always cringe when people jump into the keto diet and stop eating fruits and veggies and starting feasting on mountains of cheese and bacon," says Christie. "Veggies are critical to health, wellbeing, muscle building and a whole host of things."

A truly well-designed ketogenic diet is mainly made up of healthy fats, fruits and vegetables, and smaller quantities of healthy proteins – and our experts also note that prebiotics and probiotics are an essential part of these diets too. When looked at then, the keto diet becomes a superfood diet made of nature's medicine, including cancer-fighting antioxidants and polyphenols.

It's no wonder a healthful, well-designed ketogenic diet is linked to health benefits like the prevention of cancer.

3. Keto calls for intermittent fasting, and intermittent fasting is the ideal anti-inflammatory protocol.

While not all iterations of the keto diet require intermittent fasting, the two often go together, and for good reason: intermittent fasting may be one of the best anti-inflammatory practices of all, thus making it ideal for treating or preventing cancer.

To understand just why intermittent fasting is so good for gut health, Zupec-Kania compares it to mediation.

"Everyone stresses the concept of why meditation is good for our mental health," says Zupec-Kania. "That's been well published and recommended by standard doctors everywhere. So, I like to use that for a metaphor with what goes on in your gut - it's like meditation for your gut. It rests, it rejuvenates, and it renews. And it's so powerful that it can turn back the clock on even aging."

Studies have linked intermittent fasting to health benefits like cell repair, and one 2013 study in Current Opinion in Oncology even showed a promising link between fasting and reduced incidence of carcinogenesis and tumor growth.

"Anything in your gut triggers inflammation," says Zupec-Kania. Reducing that inflammation through intermittent fasting, especially in tandem with a well-designed ketogenic diet, may be one of the best ways to keep your body healthy and stave off the development of cancer.

Cannabis Oil/CBD

https://theuniversalplant.com/cbd-inflammation/

The body of research will no doubt continue to grow as more funding pours into this space, and as public interest continues to rise. Also, when cannabis becomes federally legal in the United States, then we will really see a large influx of research funding into the therapeutic uses of the plant.

Research around the compounds in this plant for inflammation reduction is especially important because inflammation is basically a bodily state that correlates to many life-threatening diseases. Many people's lives can be saved through proper prevention measures, and for those individuals who are deep into their issues with inflammation, they may be able to turn things around before it is too late.

What Is Inflammation?

Before we dive into the research around CBD and Hemp and Inflammation, I think it's appropriate to define what inflammation truly is. Armed with this basic understanding, you'll more firmly grasp the results of the studies I'm going to present to you today.

Inflammation is a bodily response to harmful stimuli.

Many things can cause this response in your body, which is why inflammation is more of what I would consider a "warning sign" rather than a disease itself. Like I mentioned earlier, because it is a warning sign it typically correlates with many different diseases in humans.

The major easy-to-spot signs that you have inflammation issues are: pain, swelling, soreness, fatigue, itchy skin, redness, heat, and even gut issues like Ulcerative Colitis, IBS, and diarrhea.

Inflammation is basically a generic response to a threat to your health. Your body activates your immune system as you try to fight off the "attacker." Unfortunately for most people, their habits are what causes the inflammation in the first place.

They are attacking themselves!

Bad habits like poor diet, micronutrient deficiencies, excess stress, and constant exposure to endocrine disrupting chemicals like those found in plastics, smog in the air, and even many foods, are constantly bombarding our bodies every single day, and unless you are aware of them, you're essentially just reinforcing their attack on your body.

It's no wonder inflammation is such a common thing these days, and autoimmune diseases are increasing in number every single year. We are quite literally enabling this to happen to ourselves. And unless we wake up to this reality, it will continue to happen.

Cannabidiol As An Emergent Inflammation Therapy

Inflammation has traditionally been a tricky nail to hammer for researchers when it comes to finding a therapeutic solution. The most promising area of study has involved the endocannabinoid system, namely CB1 and CB2 receptor activation which are G-protein-coupled receptor sites and the ligands that activate them.

Cannabidiol has a distinct way of interacting with the endocannabinoid system that appears very promising for therapeutic applications with relation to inflammation.1 This article will serve as an easy-to-read synopsis of much of the research in this area regarding inflammation correlated with arthritis, Type and diabetes, atherosclerosis, Alzheimer's, hypertension, metabolic syndrome, depression, and neuropathy.

Studies On The Benefits CBD and Hemp For Inflammation

Throughout this article, I will cite specific research papers next to each claim, however I think it also may be helpful for some of you who are more interested in digging deeply into this body of research, to have a specific list of research papers regarding cannabidiol and inflammation that can give you a more thorough understanding of the subject.

There are more papers out there, but this is my short list of recommended reading on the hemp and inflammation:

Cannabidiol as an emergent therapeutic strategy for lessening the impact of inflammation on oxidative stress

The endocannabinoid system: an emerging key player in inflammation

Anti-inflammatory role of cannabidiol and O-1602 in cerulein-induced acute pancreatitis in mice

Cannabinoids, endocannabinoids, and related analogs in inflammation

Cannabidiol, a non-psychotropic plant-derived cannabinoid, decreases inflammation in a murine model of acute lung injury: role for the adenosine A(2A) receptor

Cannabinoids suppress inflammatory and neuropathic pain by targeting α3 glycine receptors

Cannabidiol reduces intestinal inflammation through the control of neuroimmune axis

Diabetic retinopathy: Role of inflammation and potential therapies for anti-inflammation

Cannabidiol reduces Aβ-induced neuroinflammation and promotes hippocampal neurogenesis through PPARγ involvement

Cannabidiol attenuates high glucose-induced endothelial cell inflammatory response and barrier disruption

Vanilloid TRPV1 receptor mediates the antihyperalgesic effect of the nonpsychoactive cannabinoid, cannabidiol, in a rat model of acute inflammation

Cannabidiol attenuates cisplatin-induced nephrotoxicity by decreasing oxidative/nitrosative stress, inflammation, and cell death

Cannabinoids in clinical practice

Pure THC-V inhibits nitrite production in murine peritoneal macrophages

Cannabinoids, inflammation, and fibrosis

Amyloid proteotoxicity initiates an inflammatory response blocked by cannabinoids

Endocannabinoid 2-arachidonoylglycerol protects inflammatory insults from sulfur dioxide inhalation via cannabinoid receptors in the brain

Protective effect of CBD on hydrogen peroxide-induced apoptosis, inflammation, and oxidative stress in nucleus pulposus cells

Mechanisms of action of CBD in adoptively transferred experimental autoimmune encephalomyelitis

Hemp Extract, CBD, and Pain:

Neuropathy is caused by microglia (the most common form of cellular immune defense) activation in the brain and spinal cord, which triggers the release of the cytokines interleukin-6 (IL-6), interleukin-1β (IL-1β), and tumor necrosis factor-α (TNFα), which put into simple terms, are pro-inflammatory molecules.

The causes of neuropathic pain itself are poorly understood outside of this basic biological reaction. However, neuropathy pain is present in nearly all common forms of disease such as diabetes, cancer, autoimmune diseases, and MS.9

In a mouse model, CBD was demonstrated to alleviate heat sensitivity and allodynia (neuropathy pain) significantly.8

Two other studies demonstrated a very impressive calming of the immune system microglia/cytokine response along with promising anti-inflammatory improvements in patients with rheumatoid arthritis.9 10

CBD and Diabetes

By reducing insulin resistance and increasing insulin sensitivity, CBD was found in two separate research studies to reduce the initiation of diabetes and the development of latent diabetes in diabetes prone subjects.3 11 The super cool thing about this, is that this result was also accompanied by a shift from a pro-inflammatory cytokine response to an anti-inflammatory response.

Major effectors of β-cell death in type 1 diabetes are various free radicals and oxidant species, including NO, and infiltrating macrophages are one source of high concentrations of NO and inflammatory cytokines that further enhance NO and ROS formation.12

CBD oil has been shown in multiple studies to block ROS-induced up-regulation of surface adhesion molecules due to high blood glucose levels, which has preserved the barrier function of the endothelial cells,13 thus restricting those pesky free radicals and other oxidant species from infiltrating the β-cells.14

CBD To Help Depression and Anxiety

A large body of evidence in recent years has implicated this similar cytokine inflammatory response15 with depression in humans.16 The most convincing explanation is that the presence of excessive free radicals and oxidant species triggers the microglial cells to signal the release of the pro-inflammatory cytokines, which leads to depressive symptoms.

CBD has been reported to aid in calming this response in medical research.7

This study specifically assessed the anti-depressant and mood-elevating activity of CBD oil finding that its effect appeared to be dose dependent.17

This study posits that this anti-depressant effect of CBD oil is likely due to activation of 5-HT1A receptors in the brain.18

Cannabidiol and Anti-Pain Anti-Inflammation Applications

Research in this area of CBD and inflammation is quickly evolving, and many of these papers I've cited here have put forward some very interesting theories surrounding promising therapies for people with diseases characterized by inflammation response due to microglial cell activation and the resulting pro-inflammatory cytokine increase.

I think it is very important to also identify the actual causes of this inflammatory trigger, however countless people across the world are now in this state of poor health due to their own poor decisions (both known and unknown). It may not be their fault, but now it becomes our responsibility to do something positive to help ourselves by first calming down our inflammation response using effective natural therapies, then next we need to identify the causes of our personal inflammation and get rid of those bad habits, whether they're stress-related, nutrition-relation, or due to exposure to environmental toxins.

Cannabis Oil

Cannabis oil is an excellent cancer fighter. There has been a lot of research about cannabis oil. Maybe when the FDA figures out to make money off cannabis oil, they will research it. The problem with cannabis oil is everyone tries to make a profit off it and there is no way to know if it works.

[Cannabidiol in cancer treatment] - PubMed (nih.gov)

Cannabis was used for cancer patients as early as about 2500 years ago. Experimental studies demonstrated tumor-inhibiting activities of various cannabinoids more than 40 years ago. In view of the status of tetrahydrocannabinol (THC) as a regulated substance, non-psychotomimetic cannabidiol (CBD) is of particular importance.

Cannabis for cancer - illusion or the tip of an iceberg: a review of the evidence for the use of Cannabis and synthetic cannabinoids in oncology - PubMed (nih.gov)

A flowering plant of variegated ingredients and psychoactive qualities, Cannabis has long been used for medicinal and recreational purposes. Regulatory approvals have been gained across a broad range of palliative and therapeutic indications, and in some cases, included in standard treatment guidelines.

Sufficient evidence supports the use of Cannabis for palliative indications in oncology; however, patients should be carefully selected, guided, and followed. Promising research suggests the potent antineoplastic activity, but more data must be accrued before conclusions can be draw

[Cannabidiol in cancer treatment] - PubMed (nih.gov)

Background: Cannabis was used for cancer patients as early as about 2500 years ago. Experimental studies demonstrated tumor-inhibiting activities of various cannabinoids more than 40 years ago. In view of the status of tetrahydrocannabinol (THC) as a regulated substance, non-psychotomimetic cannabidiol (CBD) is of particular importance.

Objectives: Efficacy of pure CBD in various animal models as well as initial results (case reports) from patients.

Methods: Review of the literature on animal experiments and observations in humans.

Results: Preclinical studies, particularly recent ones, including numerous animal models of tumors, unanimously suggest the therapeutic efficacy of CBD. In isolated combination studies, synergistic effects were generally observed. In addition, CBD may potentially play a role in the palliative care of patients, especially concerning symptoms such as pain, insomnia, anxiety, and depression. Further human studies are warranted.

Clinicians' Guide to Cannabidiol and Hemp Oils - PubMed (nih.gov)

Cannabidiol (CBD) oils are low tetrahydrocannabinol products derived from Cannabis sativa that have become very popular over the past few years. Patients report relief for a variety of conditions, particularly pain, without the intoxicating adverse effects of medical marijuana. In June 2018, the first CBD-based drug, Epidiolex, was approved by the US Food and Drug Administration for treatment of rare, severe epilepsy, further putting the spotlight on CBD and hemp oils. There is a growing body of preclinical and clinical evidence to support use of CBD oils for many conditions, suggesting its potential role as another option for treating challenging chronic pain or opioid addiction. Care must be taken when directing patients toward CBD products because there is little regulation, and studies have found inaccurate labeling of CBD and tetrahydrocannabinol quantities. This article provides an overview of the scientific work on cannabinoids, CBD, and hemp oil and the distinction between marijuana, hemp, and the different components of CBD and hemp oil products. We summarize the current legal status of CBD and hemp oils in the United States and provide a guide to identifying higher-quality products so that clinicians can advise their patients on the safest and most evidence-based formulations. This review is based on a PubMed search using the terms CBD, cannabidiol, hemp oil, and medical marijuana. Articles were screened for relevance, and those with the most up-to-date information were selected for inclusion.

Melatonin

Melatonin: What You Need To Know | NCCIH (nih.gov)

What is melatonin and how does it work?

Melatonin is a hormone that your brain produces in response to darkness. It helps with the timing of your circadian rhythms (24-hour internal clock) and with sleep. Being exposed to light at night can block melatonin production.

Research suggests that melatonin plays other important roles in the body beyond sleep. However, these effects are not fully understood.

Melatonin dietary supplements can be made from animals or microorganisms, but most often they're made synthetically. The information below is about melatonin dietary supplements.

What are the health benefits of taking melatonin?

Melatonin supplements may help with certain conditions, such as jet lag, delayed sleep-wake phase disorder, some sleep disorders in children, and anxiety before and after surgery.

Jet lag
Delayed sleep-wake phase disorder (DSWPD)
Some sleep disorders in children
Anxiety before and after surgery

Is melatonin helpful for preventing or treating COVID-19?

Current research looking at the effects of melatonin on COVID-19 is only in the early stages. There are a few randomized controlled trials (studies evaluating melatonin in people) in progress. At this point, it is too soon to reach conclusions on whether melatonin is helpful for COVID-19.

Does melatonin help with cancer symptoms?

Studies of the effect of melatonin supplements on cancer symptoms or treatment-related side effects have been small and have had mixed results.

Keep in mind that unproven products should not be used to replace or delay conventional medical treatment for cancer. Also, some products can interfere with standard cancer treatments or have special risks for people who've been diagnosed with cancer. Before using any complementary health approach, including melatonin, people who have been diagnosed with cancer should talk with their health care providers to make sure that all aspects of their care work together.

Can melatonin help with insomnia?

People with insomnia have trouble falling asleep, staying asleep, or both. When symptoms last a month or longer, it's called chronic insomnia.

According to practice guidelines from the American Academy of Sleep Medicine (2017) and the American College of Physicians (2016), there's not enough strong evidence on the effectiveness or safety of melatonin supplementation for chronic insomnia to recommend its use. The American College of Physicians guidelines strongly recommend the use of cognitive behavioral therapy for insomnia (CBT-I) as an initial treatment for insomnia.

Does melatonin work for shift workers?

Shift work that involves night shifts may cause people to feel sleepy at work and make it difficult to sleep during the daytime after a shift ends.

According to two 2014 research reviews, studies on whether melatonin supplements help shift workers were generally small or inconclusive.

- The first review looked at 7 studies that included a total of 263 participants. The results suggested that (1) people taking melatonin may sleep about 24 minutes longer during the daytime, but (2) other aspects of sleep, such as time needed to fall asleep, may not change. The evidence, however, was considered to be of low quality.
- The other review looked at 8 studies (5 of which were also in the first review), with a total of 300 participants, to see whether melatonin helped promote sleep in shift workers. Six of the studies were high quality, and they had inconclusive results. The review did not make any recommendations for melatonin use in shift workers.

Is it safe to take melatonin?

For melatonin supplements, particularly at doses higher than what the body normally produces, there's not enough information yet about possible side effects to have a clear picture of overall safety. Short-term use of melatonin supplements appears to be safe for most people, but information on the long-term safety of supplementing with melatonin is lacking.

Also keep in mind:

- Interactions with medicines
- As with all dietary supplements, people who are taking medicine should consult their health care providers before using melatonin. In particular, people with epilepsy and those taking blood thinner medications need to be under medical supervision when taking melatonin supplements.
- Possible allergic reaction risk
- There may be a risk of allergic reactions to melatonin supplements.
- Safety concerns for pregnant and breastfeeding women
    - There's been a lack of research on the safety of melatonin use in pregnant or breastfeeding women.
- Safety concerns for older people
- The 2015 guidelines by the American Academy of Sleep Medicine recommend against melatonin use by people with dementia.
- Melatonin may stay active in older people longer than in younger people and cause daytime drowsiness.
- Melatonin is regulated as a dietary supplement
- In the United States, melatonin is considered a dietary supplement. This means that it's regulated less strictly by the Food and Drug Administration (FDA) than a prescription or over-the-counter drug would be. In several other countries, melatonin is available only with a prescription and is considered a drug.
- Products may not contain what's listed on the label
- Some melatonin supplements may not contain what's listed on the product label. A 2017 study tested 31 different melatonin supplements bought from grocery stores and pharmacies. For most of the supplements, the amount of melatonin in the product didn't match what was listed on the product label. Also, 26 percent of the supplements contained serotonin, a hormone that can have harmful effects even at relatively low levels.

Is melatonin safe for children?

In addition to issues mentioned above, there are some things to consider regarding melatonin's safety in children.

Melatonin supplements appear to be safe for most children for short-term use, but there aren't many studies on children and melatonin. Also, there's little information on the long-term effects of melatonin use in children. Because melatonin is a hormone, it's possible that melatonin supplements could affect hormonal development, including puberty, menstrual cycles, and overproduction of the hormone prolactin, but we don't know for sure.

Possible melatonin supplement side effects reported in children have usually been mild and have included:
- Drowsiness
- Increased bedwetting or urination in the evening
- Headache
- Dizziness
- Agitation

What are the side effects of melatonin?

A 2015 review on the safety of melatonin supplements indicated that only mild side effects were reported in various short-term studies that involved adults, surgical patients, and critically ill patients. Some of the mild side effects that were reported in the studies included:
- Headache
- Dizziness
- Nausea
- Sleepiness.

The possible long-term side effects of melatonin use are unclear.

Tips To Consider
- Remember that even though the FDA regulates dietary supplements, such as melatonin, the regulations for dietary supplements are different and less strict than those for prescription or over-the-counter drugs.
- Some dietary supplements may interact with medicines or pose risks if you have medical problems or are going to have surgery.
- If you're pregnant or nursing a child, it's especially important to see your health care provider before taking any medicine or supplement, including melatonin.
- If you use dietary supplements, such as melatonin, read and follow label instructions. "Natural" doesn't always mean "safe." For more information, see Using Dietary Supplements Wisely.
- Take charge of your health—talk with your health care providers about any complementary health approaches you use. Together, you can make shared, well-informed decisions.

For More Information

NCCIH Clearinghouse

The NCCIH Clearinghouse provides information on NCCIH and complementary and integrative health approaches, including publications and searches of Federal databases of scientific and medical literature. The Clearinghouse does not provide medical advice, treatment recommendations, or referrals to practitioners.

Toll-free in the U.S.: 1-888-644-6226
tty (for deaf and hard-of-hearing callers):
1-866-464-3615
Website: https://nccih.nih.gov/
Email: info@nccih.nih.gov(link sends e-mail)

Melatonin Facts
- Testing for melatonin – AM urine for 6-sulfatoxy melatonin.
- Peak plasma level after PO ingestion is about 1 hour. Levels sustained for 3-4 hours.
- Rapidly enters the central nervous system and crosses the blood-brain barrier.
- Exogenous melatonin does not alter the levels of any other hormones
- No negative feedback inhibition Melatonin in the treatment of cancer:
    - Direct anticancer action
    - Protects against chemo radiation damage
    - On average, the combined results of these studies showed that melatonin reduced the risk of dying by 44%.
    - The effects were consistent no matter what dose they used. ☐ None of the patients had any significant side effect from the melatonin.
    - The substantial reduction in risk of death, low adverse events reported, and low costs related to this intervention suggest great potential for melatonin in treating cancer.

Melatonin: Physiological effects in humans - PubMed (nih.gov)

Melatonin is a methoxyindole synthesized and secreted principally by the pineal gland at night under normal light/dark conditions. The endogenous rhythm of secretion is generated by the suprachiasmatic nuclei and entrained to the light/dark cycle. Light is able to either suppress or synchronize melatonin production according to the light schedule. The nyctohemeral rhythm of this hormone can be evaluated by repeated measurement of plasma or saliva melatonin or urine sulfatoxymelatonin, the main hepatic metabolite. The primary physiological function of melatonin, whose secretion adjusts to night length, is to convey information concerning the daily cycle of light and darkness to body structures. This information is used for the organisation of functions, which respond to changes in the photoperiod such as the seasonal rhythms. Seasonal rhythmicity of physiological functions in humans related to possible alteration of the melatonin message remains, however, of limited evidence in temperate areas under field conditions. Also, the daily melatonin secretion, which is a very robust biochemical signal of night, can be used for the organisation of circadian rhythms. Although functions of this hormone in humans are mainly based on correlations between clinical observations and melatonin secretion, there is some evidence that melatonin stabilizes and strengthens coupling of circadian rhythms, especially of core temperature and sleep-wake rhythms. The circadian organisation of other physiological functions depend also on the melatonin signal, for instance immune, antioxidant defences, haemostasis and glucose regulation. The difference between physiological and pharmacological effects of melatonin is not always clear but is based upon consideration of dose and not of duration of the hormone message. It is admitted that a "physiological" dose provides plasma melatonin levels in the same order of magnitude as a nocturnal peak. Since the regulating system of melatonin secretion is complex, following central and autonomic pathways, there are many pathophysiological situations where melatonin secretion can be disturbed. The resulting alteration could increase the predisposition to disease, add to the severity of symptoms or modify the course and outcome of the disorder. Since melatonin receptors display a very wide distribution in the body, putative therapeutic indications of this compound are multiple. Great advances in this field could be achieved by developing multicentre trials in a large series of patients, in order to establish efficacy of melatonin and absence of long-term toxicity.

Role of melatonin in cancer treatment - PubMed (nih.gov)

Melatonin has revealed itself to be a pleiotropic and multitasking molecule. The mechanisms that control its synthesis and the biological clock processes that modulate the circadian production of melatonin in the pineal gland have been well-characterized. A feature that characterizes melatonin is the variety of mechanisms it employs to modulate the physiology and molecular biology of cells. Research has implicated the pineal gland and melatonin in the processes of both aging and age-related diseases. The decline in the production of melatonin with age is thought to contribute to immunosenescence and potential development of neoplastic diseases. Melatonin has been shown to inhibit growth of different tumors under both in vitro and in vivo conditions. There is evidence that the administration of melatonin alone or in combination with interleukin-2 in conjunction with chemoradiotherapy and/or supportive care in cancer patients with advanced solid tumors, has been associated with improved outcomes of tumor regression and survival. Moreover, chemotherapy has been shown to be better tolerated in patients treated with melatonin.

Melatonin in Cancer Treatment: Current Knowledge and Future Opportunities (nih.gov)

Melatonin is a pleotropic molecule with numerous biological activities. Epidemiological and experimental studies have documented that melatonin could inhibit different types of cancer in vitro and in vivo. Results showed the involvement of melatonin in different anticancer mechanisms including apoptosis induction, cell proliferation inhibition, reduction in tumor growth and metastases, reduction in the side effects associated with chemotherapy and radiotherapy, decreasing drug resistance in cancer therapy, and augmentation of the therapeutic effects of conventional anticancer therapies. Clinical trials revealed that melatonin is an effective adjuvant drug to all conventional therapies. This review summarized melatonin biosynthesis, availability from natural sources, metabolism, bioavailability, anticancer mechanisms of melatonin, its use in clinical trials, and pharmaceutical formulation. Studies discussed in this review will provide a solid foundation for researchers and physicians to design and develop new therapies to treat and prevent cancer using melatonin.

Conflict of interest statement

Declaration of Competing Interest The authors declare that they have no competing interests. Melatonin is a hormone that your brain produces in response to darkness. Being exposed to light at night can block melatonin production.

Studies of the effect of melatonin supplements on cancer symptoms or treatment-related side effects have been small and have had mixed results.

Keep in mind that unproven products should not be used to replace or delay conventional medical treatment for cancer. Also, some products can interfere with standard cancer treatments or have special risks for people who've been diagnosed with cancer. Before using any complementary health approach, including melatonin, people who have been diagnosed with cancer should talk with their health care providers to make sure that all aspects of their care work together.

For melatonin supplements, particularly at doses higher than what the body normally produces, there's not enough information yet about possible side effects to have a clear picture of overall safety. Short-term use of melatonin supplements appears to be safe for most people, but information on the long-term safety of supplementing with melatonin is lacking.

Also keep in mind:
- Interactions with medicines
- As with all dietary supplements, people who are taking medicine should consult their health care providers before using melatonin. In particular, people with epilepsy and those taking blood thinner medications need to be under medical supervision when taking melatonin supplements.
- Possible allergic reaction risk

- There may be a risk of allergic reactions to melatonin supplements.
- Safety concerns for pregnant and breastfeeding women
    - There's been a lack of research on the safety of melatonin use in pregnant or breastfeeding women.
- Safety concerns for older people
- The 2015 guidelines by the American Academy of Sleep Medicine recommend against melatonin use by people with dementia.
- Melatonin may stay active in older people longer than in younger people and cause daytime drowsiness.
- Melatonin is regulated as a dietary supplement
- In the United States, melatonin is considered a dietary supplement. This means that it's regulated less strictly by the Food and Drug Administration (FDA) than a prescription or over-the-counter drug would be. In several other countries, melatonin is available only with a prescription and is considered a drug.
- Products may not contain what's listed on the label
- Some melatonin supplements may not contain what's listed on the product label. A 2017 study tested 31 different melatonin supplements bought from grocery stores and pharmacies. For most of the supplements, the amount of melatonin in the product didn't match what was listed on the product label. Also, 26 percent of the supplements contained serotonin, a hormone that can have harmful effects even at relatively low levels.

A 2015 review on the safety of melatonin supplements indicated that only mild side effects were reported in various short-term studies that involved adults, surgical patients, and critically ill patients. Some of the mild side effects that were reported in the studies included:
- Headache
- Dizziness
- Nausea
- Sleepiness.

The possible long-term side effects of melatonin use are unclear.

Melatonin and its derivative disrupt cancer stem-like phenotypes of lung cancer cells via AKT downregulation - PubMed (nih.gov)

Cancer stem cells (CSCs), a small subpopulation of tumor cells, have properties of self-renewal and multipotency, which drive cancer progression and resistance to current treatments. Compounds potentially targeting **CSCs** have been recently developed. This study shows how **melatonin**, an endogenous hormone synthesized by the pineal gland, and its derivative suppress **CSC**-like phenotypes of human non-small cell lung cancer cell lines. The effects of MLT and its derivative, acetyl **melatonin** (ACT), on CSC-like phenotypes were investigated using assays for anchorage-independent growth, three-dimensional spheroid formation, scratch wound healing ability, and CSC marker and upstream protein signaling expression. Enriched CSC spheroids were used to confirm the effect of both compounds on lung cancer cells. MLT and ACT inhibited CSC-like behaviors by suppression of colony and spheroid formation in NSCLC cell lines. Their effects on spheroid formation were confirmed in CSC-enriched H460 cells. CSC markers, CD133 and ALDH1A1, were depleted by both compounds. The behavior and factors associated to epithelial-mesenchymal transition, as indicated by cell migration and the protein vimentin, were also decreased by MLT and ACT. Mechanistically, MLT and ACT decreased the expression of stemness proteins Oct-4, Nanog, and β-catenin by reducing active AKT (phosphorylated AKT). Suppression of the AKT pathway was not mediated through melatonin receptors. This study demonstrates a novel role, and its underlying mechanism, for MLT and its derivative ACT in suppression of CSC-like phenotypes in NSCLC cells, indicating that they are potential candidates for lung cancer treatment.

High Dose Melatonin
[The Therapeutic Effects of High-Dose Melatonin Administration - Antiaging Systems (antiaging-systems.com)](antiaging-systems.com)
Written by [Tresguerres, M.D., Ph.D., Jesus](Tresguerres)
This article reviews the effects of high-dose melatonin administration on several diseases. Experimental studies performed over more than 20 years have shown that oxidative stress and **inflammation** increase in nearly all tissues with many degenerative diseases or aging. We have measured several parameters related to oxidative stress, **inflammation, and apoptosis** both in several models of aging and after ischemia in the liver or brain. The effect of treatment with melatonin has been evaluated showing a significant reduction of **inflammation**, **apoptosis** markers and parameters related to oxidative stress, in several tissues. **Inflammations**, as well as oxidative stress and **apoptosis** markers were increased also in degenerative diseases like diabetes, hypertension, or Parkinson disease so treatment with melatonin should also have very positive effects.

When the skin is submitted to ionizing radiation like radiotherapy a marked release of free radicals inducing inflammation and oxidative stress is obtained giving rise to radiodermatitis. All of the above-mentioned parameters have been also shown to be increased in the skin. Melatonin treatment was able to reduce those markers and oxidative stress preventing the appearance of radiodermatitis.

The conclusion is that melatonin administration exerts beneficial effects against age- or degenerative diseases induced changes in several tissues and functions.

Melatonin, an indole hormone secreted by the pineal gland, is a substance closely related to biological rhythms and has been used since decades for the induction of sleep and the treatment of jet lag. In addition to its role as a chrono biotic hormone, melatonin is a ubiquitous direct free radical scavenger and an important indirect antioxidant. Moreover, melatonin is a small, lipophilic, and hydrophilic molecule, what allows it to easily cross biological barriers and membranes, and diffuse throughout cell compartments, reaching the place where the free radicals and reactive species are generated in all tissues: the mitochondria.

Besides to these direct scavenging actions, melatonin also stimulates a host of endogenous antioxidant enzymes, including Superoxide Dismutase (SOD), glutathione peroxidase (GPx) and glutathione reductase (GRd), and inhibits the activity of Nitric oxide synthase (NOS) thus making possible to effectively fight against free radicals but also against **inflammation, apoptosis** and in several age associated diseases.

Dosing
- Only red lights in the bedroom.
- Prevention: 180 mg about 30 minutes before bedtime.
- Treatment: 60 mg 3-6x/day
- 300mg two hours before PET/CT
- Melatonin Max – 60 mg pure capsules (www.scientifichealthsolutions.com)
- **Melatonin powder – www.purebulk.com**
  - Zero contraindications

Melatonin at high doses protects against cancer | Neolife (neolifeclinic.com) by Neolife on 22 May 2018 in Hormonal balance, Prevention and Anti-aging

---

Therapy - An Ideal Adjuvant Anti-Cancer Therapy (riordanclinic.org)
- Produced and released in pineal gland in darkness. Immediately suppressed by all light but red light.
  - Not a soporific. You can take it during the day, as well as at bedtime, without any adverse effect.
- Side effects: no serious side effects. Some patients report sleep disturbances and AM sleepiness.

- Dr. Pierpaoli, one of the world's leading melatonin researchers, has successfully used daily dosages ranging from 0.1 to 200 mg. That's a 2,000-fold difference between the lowest dose and the highest! Studies on mice show that even at astronomical doses of 300 mg per day for two years, there were no side effects.

Basic mechanisms involved in the anti-cancer effects of melatonin.
Melatonin has oncostatic properties in a wide variety of tumors.
- Mitochondrial stimulant.
- Regulation of estrogen receptor expression and transactivation.
- Modulation of the enzymes involved in the local synthesis of estrogens.
  ☐ Modulation of cell cycle and induction of apoptosis.
- Inhibition of telomerase activity
- Inhibition of metastasisBasic mechanisms involved in the anti-cancer effects of melatonin.

Mediavilla MD1, Sanchez-Barcelo EJ, et al. Curr Med Chem 2010;17(36):4462-81.
• Direct anti-neoplastic effects.
• Decreases cell proliferation at low concentrations.
• Direct cytotoxic effect occurs with high concentrations
• Stimulation of cell differentiation
• Induction of **apoptosis**
• Anti-angiogenesis
• A synergistic effect has been found in several cancer types when it is administered in combination with chemotherapy.

Cancer metastasis: Mechanisms of inhibition by melatonin.
Due to the broad range of melatonin's actions, the mechanisms underlying its ability to interfere with metastases are numerous.
- melatonin reduces the uptake of glucose and modifies the expression of GLUT1 transporter in prostate cancer cells.
- Melatonin reduces endothelin-1 expression and secretion in colon cancer cells through the inactivation of FoxO-1 and NF-$\varkappa\beta$.
- Endothelin-1 (ET-1) is a peptide that acts as a survival factor in colon cancer, inducing cell proliferation, protecting carcinoma cells from apoptosis, and promoting angiogenesis."
- The data presented show that melatonin inhibits edn-1 mRNA expression, the first step in ET-1 synthesis."

- In conclusion, melatonin may be useful in treating colon carcinoma in which the activation of ET-1 plays a role in tumor growth and progression."

Melatonin as a potential anticarcinogen for non-small-cell lung cancer. Ma Z, Yang Y, Fan C. Oncotarget. 2016 Jul 19;7(29):46768-46784
- Melatonin exerts pleiotropic anticancer effects against a variety of cancer types.
- Herein, we review the correlation between the disruption of the melatonin rhythm and NSCLC incidence.
- We also evaluate the evidence related to the effects of melatonin in inhibiting lung carcinogenesis. Special focus is placed on the oncostatic effects of melatonin, including antiproliferation, induction of apoptosis, inhibition of invasion and metastasis, and enhancement of immunomodulation.
- We suggest the drug synergy of melatonin with radio- or chemotherapy for NSCLC could prove to be useful.
- Melatonin as a treatment for gastrointestinal cancer: a review. Xin Z, Jiang S, Jiang P. J Pineal Res. 2015 May;58(4):375-87.
- The ability of melatonin to inhibit gastrointestinal cancer is substantial."
- In this review, we first clarify the relationship between the disruption of the melatonin rhythm and gastrointestinal cancer.
- The mechanisms through which melatonin exerts its antigastrointestinal cancer actions are explained, including inhibition of proliferation, invasion, metastasis, and angiogenesis, and promotion of apoptosis and cancer immunity."
- We discuss the drug synergy effects and the role of melatonin receptors involved in the growth-inhibitory effects on gastrointestinal cancer.
- The information compiled here serves as a comprehensive reference for the anti-gastrointestinal cancer actions of melatonin that have been identified to date.

Melatonin uses in oncology: breast cancer prevention and reduction of the side effects of chemotherapy and radiation. Sanchez-Barcelo EJ, Mediavilla MD, Expert Opin Investig Drugs. 2012 Jun;21(6):819-31.

Because of its SERM (selective estrogen receptor modulators) and SEEM (selective estrogen enzyme modulators) properties, and its virtual absence of contraindications, melatonin could be an excellent adjuvant with the drugs currently used for breast cancer prevention (antiestrogens and antiaromatases)."

- The antioxidant actions also make melatonin a suitable treatment to reduce oxidative stress associated with chemotherapy, especially with anthracyclines, and radiotherapy."
- Melatonin's anti-estrogenic properties are especially useful for breast cancer prevention in cases of obesity, steroid hormone treatment or chrono disruption by exposure to light at night. Protective and sensitive effects of melatonin combined with adriamycin on ER+ (estrogen receptor) breast cancer.

Ma C, Li LX, Zhang Y, Xiang C, Eur J Gynaecol Oncol. 2015;36(2):197-202.

- ER+ breast cancer rat model was established and then rats were randomly divided into five different groups as follows: control group, Diss group, Adriamycin (ADM) group, MLT group, and MLT combined with adriamycin (M+A) group.
- Tumor weights were significantly lighter in M+A group than those in ADM group ($p < 0.05$). Under optical and electro-microscopy, tumor cell apoptosis was obviously increased in MLT group, and tumor cell injury was more severe in M+A group than that in ADM group.
- Decreased E-cadherin expression in cancer cells increases proliferation, invasion, and/or metastasis. Expression of E-cadherin was higher in MLT group and M+A group than that in other groups. ꓘ MLT group had the highest one month survival rate (100%), there was the poorest life quality in ADM group, but the best life quality in MLT.
- MLT could enhance the sensitivity of tumor to ADM in vivo and improve patient's life quality."

Physiological and pharmacological concentrations of melatonin protect against cisplatin-induced acute renal injury. J. Pineal Res. 2002 Oct;33(3):161-6.

- Acute tubular necrosis is a major side effect of cisplatin
- Melatonin is a direct free radical scavenger and indirect antioxidant."
- We investigated the effects of melatonin on cisplatin-induced changes of renal malondialdehyde (MDA), a lipid peroxidation product, and blood urea nitrogen (BUN) and serum creatine (Cr). The morphological changes in kidney were also examined using light microscopy.
- Melatonin administration either before or after CDDP injection caused significant decreases in MDA.
- The morphological damage to the kidney induced by cisplatin was reversed by melatonin.
- The results show that pharmacological and physiological concentrations of melatonin reduce cisplatin-induced renal injury."

Melatonin as a radioprotective agent: a review. Vijayalaxmi, Reiter RJ, et al. Int J Radiat Oncol Biol Phys. 2004 Jul 1;59(3):639-53.
- Melatonin is both a direct and indirect free radical scavenger.
- The radical scavenging ability of melatonin works via electron donation to detoxify hydroxyl radical.
- Ionizing radiation results in the production of hydroxyl radical.
- The results from many in vitro and in vivo investigations have confirmed that melatonin protects mammalian cells from the toxic effects of ionizing radiation.
- Furthermore, several clinical reports indicate that melatonin administration, either alone or in combination with traditional radiotherapy, results in a favorable efficacy: toxicity ratio during the treatment of human cancers. Melatonin for Prevention of Breast Radiation Dermatitis: A Phase II, Prospective, Double-Blind Randomized Trial.

Ben-David MA, Elkayam R, et al. Isr Med Assoc J. 2016 Mar-Apr;18(3-4):188-92.
- Radiation-induced dermatitis is commonly seen during radiotherapy for breast cancer.
- randomized, placebo-controlled double-blind study, patients randomly allocated to topical cream twice daily use during radiation treatment and 2 weeks following the end of radiotherapy.
- Grade 1-2 acute radiation dermatitis was 59% vs. 90% in the melatonin group.
- Patients treated with melatonin-containing emulsion experienced significantly reduced radiation dermatitis compared to patients receiving placebo.

Melatonin is produced in the pineal gland, located deep in the brain and which was considered a possible receptacle for the soul in the early stages of neuroanatomy.

This molecule has been the subject of numerous studies since the 80s and, little by little, we've been finding out the surprising effects it has. These are not just limited to sleep, but throughout the body. We could even stretch to say that sleep improvement plays a secondary role to the rest of the benefits.

Dr. Iván Moreno – Neolife Medical Team

Now we're going to look at the different benefits melatonin has.

This recently discovered molecule (1958), has been the subject of numerous studies since the 80s and, little by little, we've been finding out the surprising effects it has. These are not just limited to sleep, but throughout the body. We could even stretch to say that sleep improvement plays a secondary role to the rest of the benefits.

Melatonin is produced in the pineal gland, located deep in the brain and which was considered a possible receptacle for the soul in the early stages of neuroanatomy. There is melatonin in many species of animals and plants, which shows its basic importance in the metabolism of living beings.

High concentrations of melatonin have been found in the retina, gastrointestinal tract, bone marrow, skin, and other tissues. We can therefore deduce that it may have an influence on other physiological functions through local secretion and that, far from being just a sleeping aid, melatonin has multiple effects throughout the body, including:

- Regulating the different biological clocks of the body: biological neural clocks are adjusted in cycles more or less approximate to the duration of the day (22-26 hours), but the other daily cycles of the organism such as hepatic metabolism, renal, oxidative stress, body temperature and muscle toning have less accurate clocks, so they require internal synchronization. That is why when we suffer jetlag, we're not only tired, but we feel almost sick – our body does not work properly.
- Control of oxidative stress: melatonin plays a key role in promoting the excellent health of mitochondria and an adequate control of oxidative stress.
- Prevention of dementia.
- Maintenance of the optimal neuronal state.
- Others…

The secretion of melatonin is influenced by external light through the optic nerve. This means nature allows us to synchronize with seasonal changes.

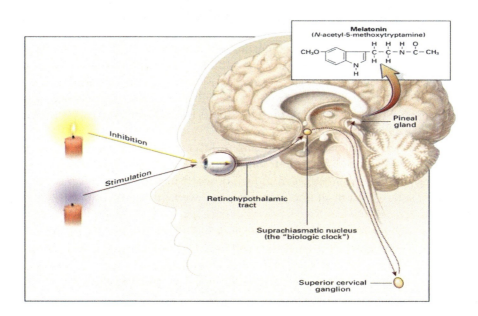

Illustration 1- Free access on Pubmed central, courtesy of the Journal of Clinical Sleep Medicine).

Each of us has a particular predisposition for melatonin secretion, the most frequent being the average that begins producing melatonin at around 8:00 in the evening and peaks about 2:00-3:00 in the morning.

Quite often we find, when studying the secretion profile, a lack of coordination and insufficient secretion.

These phase imbalances and deficits in the total effect of melatonin cause the appearance of chrono biotic rhythm alterations, imbalance, and oxidative stress, etc.

As we age, melatonin secretion drops in quality, resulting in imbalances of the circadian cycles and quantity thereof (figure attached).

Although the doses normally found in supplements are around 2mg, these doses are too small to reach all tissues and serve the different purposes that melatonin has. In addition, in case of using an incorrect dose we can produce the opposite effect (insomnia or de-regulation), which is why taking melatonin supplements without measuring precisely normally only goes well for some people while others report insomnia and discomfort.

At ***Neolife*** we advocate taking high doses of melatonin, which have the maximum beneficial effects, but at a personalized dose and at a specific time which will be most beneficial (and which will avoid side effects). For this reason, in collaboration with the International Institute of Melatonin, we conducted studies of melatonin profiles and oxidative stress to be able to prescribe melatonin and antioxidants properly.

Age Management Medicine Group

Recently at the annual meeting of the AMMG in Orlando, Florida, attended by part of the Neolife medical team, results from several studies were presented which showed an antineoplastic effect from high doses of melatonin. In this post we want to review some of the most important ideas that were presented:

- There is no such thing as "high doses" of melatonin. Melatonin has been shown to be extremely safe and toxic levels of it have not yet been shown. This does not mean that we can take high doses without conducting a previous study, as even if we do not have to avoid the toxicity, we still need to pay attention to the balance of the system.
- Exposure to blue spectrum light is the most related to the secretion of melatonin. To secrete melatonin, you do not need to sleep, you only need to be in the dark. Professor Ritter went on to say that light at night "is a drug" in relation to the harmful effects it has. This is of extreme importance as the secretion of melatonin and the preparation for an adequate night's rest begins hours before going to bed (normally at 08:00pm). Maintaining good sleep hygiene and adapting screens to avoid blue light is essential to preserve our melatonin secretion as long as possible.
- Melatonin and all its metabolites have a powerful effect by capturing free radicals, which are highly toxic and damage DNA, leading to degenerative, autoinflammatory and oncological diseases. It has been seen in different studies that there is a higher incidence of cancer in workers on night shift, or with alterations in the important hourly rhythms (many transoceanic journeys). In fact, light at night is included as a carcinogen by the World Health Organization.

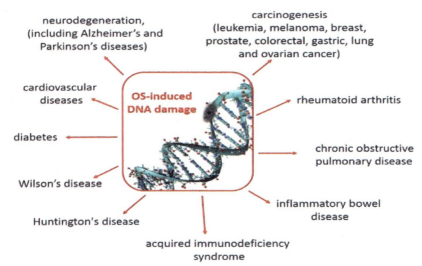

Illustration 4- Professor Russel J. Reiter. High Dose Melatonin. AMMG, April 28th, 2018, Orlando.

• There is strong scientific evidence that shows that **tumors** appear, develop, and **metastasize** more easily in subjects exposed to night light that prevents correct melatonin secretion.
• Melatonin inhibits many of the mechanisms that **cancer** cells use (Hanahan, 2011) and improves sensitivity to chemotherapy.

Following this excellent presentation and reviewing the relationship of melatonin with the appearance of **tumors**, specifically the breast, in greater depth we have found important scientific evidence that supports this relationship in human studies, showing a clear benefit in prevention and even by adding melatonin to the oncological treatment of breast tumors.

In an extensive review published in the journal Critical Reviews in Oncology last year, it was concluded that there is considerable evidence to support the multiple **tumor** suppressive effects of melatonin, showing a protective effect against **chemotherapy** and **antitumor** of melatonin, especially through its anti-gonadotropin and antiestrogenic effect on the breast tumor.

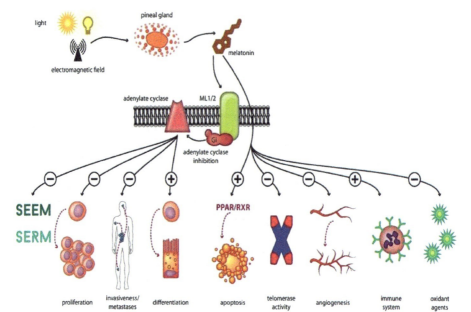

Illustration 5- Antitumor effects of melatonin. Image courtesy of the journal Critical Reviews in Oncology and Hematology, freely accessible (1)

Due to its low toxicity even in high doses and the full range of benefits that it seems to have shown, melatonin can be considered as a complementary therapy to usual chemo and radiotherapy and in prevention of breast cancer in women with a history of risk or mammary fibrocystic disease.

So then, beyond the benefits for quality of sleep, melatonin is a true antiaging molecule, while allowing vital systems to continue optimum functioning and delaying the appearance of diseases – exactly what Age Management medicine and Neolife are about.

IP-6

Phytic Acid: From Antinutritional to Multiple Protection Factor of Organic Systems - PubMed (nih.gov)

Several studies have shown the benefits of natural antioxidants on health and food preservation. Phytic acid (IP6) is a natural antioxidant that is found mainly in cereals and vegetables and, for a long period of time, was considered an antinutritional factor. However, in vitro, and in vivo studies have demonstrated its beneficial effects in the prevention and treatment of several pathological conditions and cancer. Despite the numerous benefits of IP6, the signs and intracellular interactions mediated by this antioxidant remain poorly understood. This review describes the main chemical and biological aspects of IP6, as well as its actions in the prevention and treatment of various diseases.

[IP6: a novel anti-cancer agent - PubMed (nih.gov)](#)

IP6: A novel anti-cancer agent
[A M Shamsuddin](#), [I Vucenik](#), [K E Cole](#)

Inositol hexaphosphate (InsP6 or IP6) is ubiquitous. At 10 microM to 1 mM concentrations, IP6 and its lower phosphorylated forms (IP(1-5)) as well as inositol (Ins) are contained in most mammalian cells, wherein they are important in regulating vital cellular functions such as signal transduction, cell proliferation and differentiation. A striking anti-cancer action of IP6 has been demonstrated both in vivo and in vitro, which is based on the hypotheses that exogenously administered IP6 may be internalized, dephosphorylated to IP(1-5), and inhibit cell growth. There is additional evidence that Ins alone may further enhance the anti-cancer effect of IP6. Besides decreasing cellular proliferation, IP6 also causes differentiation of malignant cells often resulting in a reversion to normal phenotype. These data strongly point towards the involvement of signal transduction pathways, cell cycle regulatory genes, differentiation genes, oncogenes and perhaps, tumor suppressor genes in bringing about the observed anti-neoplastic action of IP6.

https://pubmed.ncbi.nlm.nih.gov/17044765/

Protection against cancer by dietary IP6 and inositol
Ivana Vucenik 1, AbulKalam M Shamsuddin
Affiliations expand
PMID: 17044765 DOI: 10.1207/s15327914nc5502_1
Abstract

Inositol hexaphosphate (**IP(6)**) is a naturally occurring polyphosphorylated carbohydrate, abundantly present in many plant sources and in certain high-fiber diets, such as cereals and legumes. In addition to being found in plants, **IP(6)** is contained in almost all mammalian cells, although in much smaller amounts, where it is important in regulating vital cellular functions such as signal transduction, cell proliferation, and differentiation. For a long time, **IP(6)** has been recognized as a natural antioxidant. Recently **IP(6)** has received much attention for its role in **cancer** prevention and control of experimental tumor growth, progression, and metastasis. In addition, **IP(6)** possesses other significant benefits for human health, such as the ability to enhance immune system, prevent pathological calcification and kidney stone formation, lower elevated serum cholesterol, and reduce pathological platelet activity. In this review we show the efficacy and discuss some of the molecular mechanisms that govern the action of this dietary agent. Exogenously administered **IP(6)** is rapidly taken up into cells and dephosphorylated to lower inositol phosphates, which further affect signal transduction pathways resulting in cell cycle arrest. A striking anticancer action of **IP(6)** was demonstrated in different experimental models. In addition to reducing cell proliferation, **IP(6)** also induces differentiation of malignant cells. Enhanced immunity and antioxidant properties also contribute to tumor cell destruction. Preliminary studies in humans show that **IP(6)** and inositol, the precursor molecule of **IP(6)**, appear to enhance the **anticancer** effect of conventional chemotherapy, control cancer metastases, and improve quality of life. Because it is abundantly present in regular diet, efficiently absorbed from the gastrointestinal tract, and safe, **IP(6)** + inositol holds great promise in our strategies for **cancer** prevention and therapy. There is clearly enough evidence to justify the initiation of full-scale clinical trials in humans.

https://pubmed.ncbi.nlm.nih.gov/8669811/

IP6-induced growth inhibition and differentiation of HT-29 human colon cancer cells: involvement of intracellular inositol phosphates
G Y Yang 1, A M Shamsuddin
Affiliations expand
PMID: 8669811
Abstract
Inositol hexaphosphate (InsP6 or **IP6**) ubiquitous in plants and animals is not only a natural antioxidant but may also be the precursor/storage of intracellular inositol phosphates, important for various cellular functions. A novel **anti-tumor** action of InsP6 was demonstrated in models of experimental colon and mammary carcinogenesis in vivo. We now show its effects on growth and differentiation of HT-29 human colon carcinoma cells in vitro. A dose- and time-dependent (0.33-20 mM

InsP6 and 1-6 days treatment) growth inhibition was observed as tested by MTT-incorporation assay. The inhibition was statistically significant ($p < 0.05$) at 1 mM concentration as early as first day after treatment and continued up to 6 days. DNA-synthesis was also suppressed by InsP6 and significantly inhibited as early as 6 h after treatment at 1 mM concentration ($p < 0.05$) and continued to 48 h ($p < 0.01$). The expression of proliferation marker PCNA was down-regulated ($p < 0.05$) by InsP6 (1 and 5 mM) after 48 h of treatment. To investigate the mechanism of action of InsP6 the intracellular phosphatases (including phytase) were inhibited by F to slow down the dephosphorylation of InsP6. Ion-exchange chromatographic separation of intracellular inositol phosphates demonstrated an 84-98% decrease of Ins, InsP1 and InsP2 InsP3 was reduced by 39% and InsP4 and InsP5 by 21% and 13% respectively, whereas intracellular InsP6 was increased by 24.6% at 5 min following 3H-InsP6. Since neither the rate of uptake of 3H-InsP6 was unaffected, nor was the efficacy of growth inhibition altered by F inhibition of phytase, data suggest that contrary to the popular misconception, phytase plays no role in influencing the anti-neoplastic action of InsP6. Alkaline phosphatase activity (brush border enzyme, associated with absorptive cell differentiation), increased following 1 and 5 mM InsP6 treatment for 1-6 days. The expression of a mucin antigen associated with goblet cell differentiation and defined by the monoclonal antibody CMU10 was augmented ($p < 0.0001$) by InsP6. The tumor mucin marker Gal-GalNAc, expressed by precancer and cancer of colon, but not by the normal cells showed a time-dependent biphasic change by InsP6; an increased expression after 1 day of treatment followed by suppression after 2 days suggest progression of mucin synthesis and differentiation of cancer cells with reversion to normal phenotype. Because the tumor marker Gal-GalNAc is a) easily detected in rectal mucin of patients with colonic cancer and **precancer** with high sensitivity and specificity, and b) suppressed by InsP6 treatment, it can be used to monitor the efficacy of chemoprevention by InsP6 or other such agents. Since InsP6 a natural dietary ingredient of cereals and legumes, inhibits growth and induces terminal differentiation of HT-29 cancer cells, it is an excellent candidate for adjuvant **chemotherapy and prevention of cancer**.

https://pubmed.ncbi.nlm.nih.gov/10625949/

Metabolism and cellular functions of IP6: a review
A M Shamsuddin 1
Affiliations expand
PMID: 10625949
Abstract

Inositol hexaphosphate (**IP6**) has a demonstrably effective **anti-cancer** action against a variety of experimental tumors. However, the mechanisms of its actions are yet to be completely discerned. Studies in my laboratory have shown that **IP6** is rather rapidly absorbed by rats in vivo. Ion exchange chromatography demonstrates the presence of inositol and IP1-6 in gastric epithelial cells as early as within 1 h of intragastric 3H-IP6 administration. The metabolized IP6, in the form of inositol and IP1 is transported via plasma and reaches distant organs as well as tumors. In rats, the urinary metabolites of **IP6** are inositol and IP1. However, in humans 1-3% of total administered **IP6** is excreted in the urine as **IP6**; the level shows a normal oscillation between 0.5-6 mg/L [F. Grases et al]. Investigations of the uptake and metabolism by a variety of **cancer** cell lines in vitro also demonstrate an instantaneous absorption of **IP6**. The rate and pattern at which **IP6** is metabolized by **cancer** cells varies depending on the cell type. Intracellular inositols accumulated mostly (80-97%) in the cytosol as inositol and IP1-6. **IP6** treatment of all the cell lines tested so far demonstrates that it is cytostatic and not cytotoxic. Along with inhibition of cell proliferation, there is enhanced differentiation of malignant cells to a more mature phenotype, often resulting in reversion to normal. Studies of the expression of **tumor** suppressor gene demonstrate up-regulation of wild type p53 and down-regulation of the mutant form. Since p53-mediated cell cycle arrest may be the direct result of induction of WAF-1 gene (p21WAF-1/CIP1), our studies demonstrate that **IP6** up-regulates the expression of p21WAF-1/CIP1 in a dose-dependent manner. These data strongly point towards the involvement of signal transduction pathways, cell cycle regulatory genes, differentiation genes, oncogenes and perhaps, **tumor** suppressor genes in bringing about the observed anti-neoplastic action of **IP6**.

IP-6 are contained in most mammalian cells, wherein they are important in regulating vital cellular functions such as signal transduction, cell proliferation and differentiation. A striking **anti-cancer** action of IP6 has been demonstrated both in vivo and in vitro. IP-6, inositol hex phosphate, is a vitamin-like substance. It is found in humans, animals, and many plants, especially cereals, nuts, and legumes. It can also be made in a laboratory. Some people use IP-6 to treat and prevent **cancer**, to reduce side effects of cancer treatment, for anemia, diabetes, and many other conditions, but there is no good scientific evidence to support these uses. In manufacturing, IP-6 is added to food to keep it from spoiling. There is additional evidence that Ins alone may further enhance the anti-cancer effect of IP-6. Besides decreasing cellular proliferation, IP6 also causes differentiation of malignant cells often resulting in a reversion to normal phenotype. Several studies have shown the benefits of natural antioxidants on health and food preservation. IP-6 is a natural antioxidant that is found mainly in cereals and vegetables and, for a long period of time, was considered an antinutritional factor. However, in vitro, and in vivo studies have demonstrated its beneficial effects in the prevention and treatment of several pathological conditions and cancer. Despite the numerous benefits of IP-6, the signs and intracellular interactions mediated by this antioxidant remain poorly understood. This review describes the main chemical and biological aspects of IP-6, as well as its actions in the prevention and treatment of various diseases.

Photos

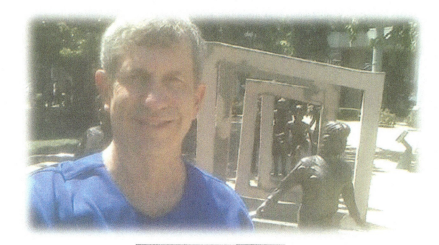

Before Radiation

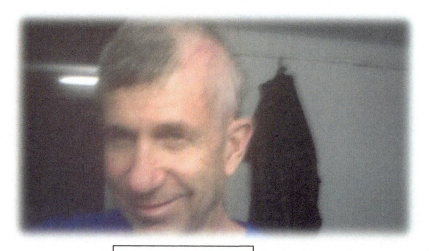

During Radiation

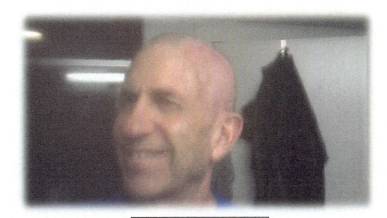

During Radiation

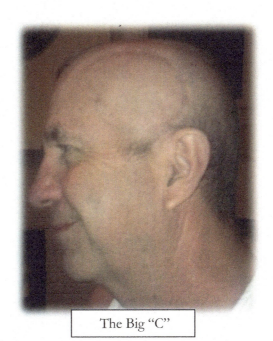

The Big "C"

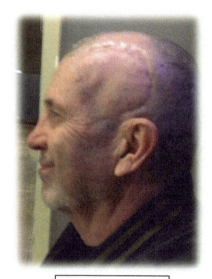

The Big "C"

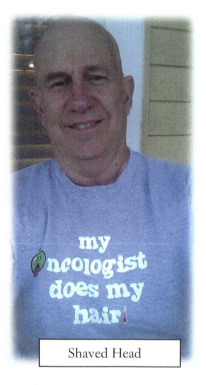

Shaved Head

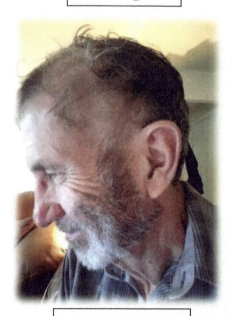

November 2018

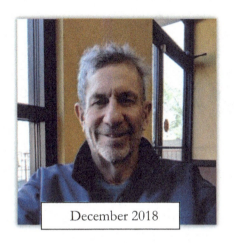

December 2018

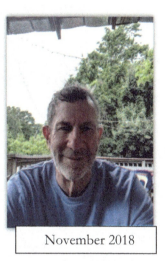

November 2018

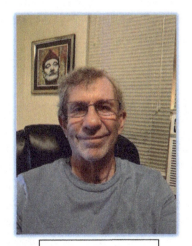

June 1, 2020

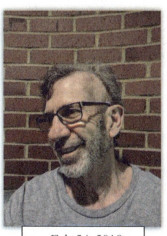

Feb 24, 2018

8/10/2014 Mississippi River

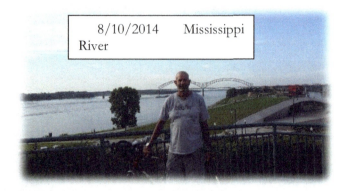

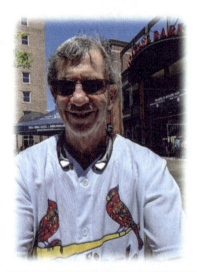

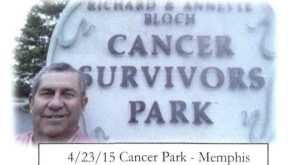

4/23/15 Cancer Park - Memphis

4/29/18 Redbird's Stadium

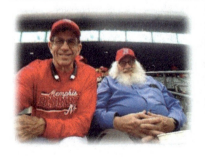

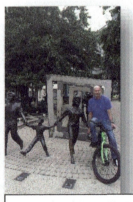

10/26/13 Dallas Cancer Park

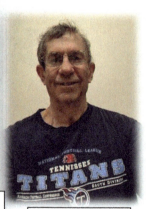

7/29/19

Cancer Parks

There are Cancer Parks in numerous cities. This one is in Memphis, Tennessee. I have seen Cancer Parks in Dallas, Texas and New Orleans, Louisiana.

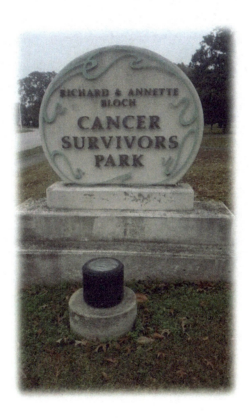

The maze represents cancer. The people coming into the maze are terrified. The people coming out of the maze are relieved

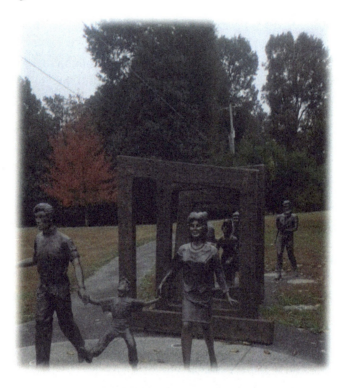

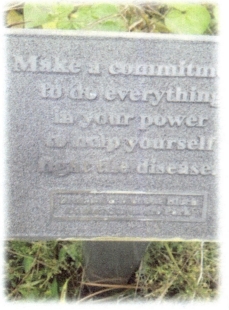

Make a commitment to do everything in your power to help yourself fight the disease

Cancer is the most curable of all chronic diseases

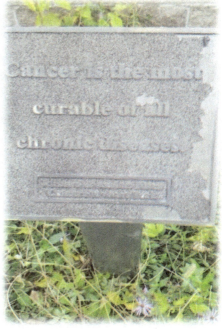

Knowledge: Knowledge is a cancer patient's best friend. The more you know about your disease the better your chances are of beating it. Find out everything you can about your disease. Knowledge heals, ignorance kills. Read the book *Fighting Cancer*. available free from 800-433-0464

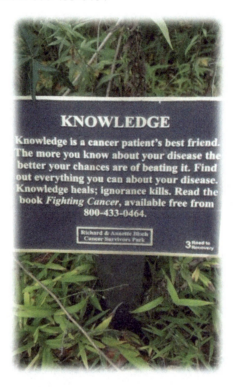

Stem Cells vs Cancer Stem Cells From Wikipedia

I am going to try and explain the differences and similarities of Stem Cells and Cancer Stem Cells. A lot of people think they are the same. They are not the same. Let's first look at Stem Cells as Wikipedia defines it.

Stem Cells
From Wikipedia, the free encyclopedia

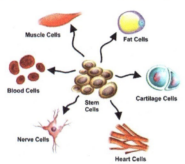

Stem cells are cells that can differentiate into other types of cells and can also divide in self-renewal to produce more of the same type of stem cells.

Telomerase is active in normal stem cells.

In mammals, there are two broad types of stem cells: embryonic stem cells, which are isolated from the inner cell mass of blastocysts in early embryonic development, and adult stem cells, which are found in various tissues of fully developed mammals. In adult organisms, stem cells and progenitor cells act as a repair system for the body, replenishing adult tissues. In a developing embryo, stem cells can differentiate into all the specialized cells—ectoderm, endoderm, and mesoderm (see induced pluripotent stem cells)—but also maintain the normal turnover of regenerative organs, such as blood, skin, or intestinal tissues.

There are three known accessible sources of autologous adult stem cells in humans: bone marrow, adipose tissue, and blood. Stem cells can also be taken from umbilical cord blood just after birth. Of all stem cell therapy types, autologous harvesting involves the least risk.

Adult stem cells are frequently used in various medical therapies (e.g., bone marrow transplantation). Stem cells can now be artificially grown and transformed (differentiated) into specialized cell types with characteristics consistent with cells of various tissues such as muscles or nerves. Embryonic cell lines and autologous embryonic stem cells generated through somatic cell nuclear transfer or dedifferentiation have also been proposed as promising candidates for future therapies. Research into stem cells grew out of findings by Ernest A. McCulloch and James E. Till at the University of Toronto in the 1960s.

Wikipedia Defines Cancer Stem Cells

Cancer Stem Cells
From Wikipedia, the free encyclopedia

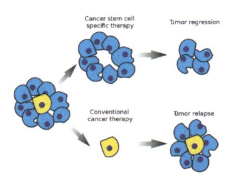

Peter Znamenskiy 2

Cancer stem cells (CSCs) are cancer cells (found within tumors or hematological cancers) that possess characteristics associated with normal stem cells, specifically the ability to give rise to all cell types found in a particular cancer sample. CSCs are therefore tumorigenic (tumor-forming), perhaps in contrast to other non-tumorigenic cancer cells. CSCs may generate tumors through the stem cell processes of self-renewal and differentiation into multiple cell types. Such cells are hypothesized to persist in tumors as a distinct population and cause relapse and metastasis by giving rise to new tumors. Therefore, development of specific therapies targeted at CSCs holds hope for improvement of survival and quality of life of cancer patients, especially for patients with metastatic disease.

Existing cancer treatments have mostly been developed based on animal models, where therapies able to promote tumor shrinkage were deemed effective. However, *animals do not provide a complete model of human disease. In particular, in mice, whose life spans do not exceed two years, tumor relapse is difficult to study.*

The efficacy of cancer treatments is, in the initial stages of testing, often measured by the ablation fraction of tumor mass (fractional kill). As CSCs form a small proportion of the tumor, this may not necessarily select for drugs that act specifically on the stem cells. *The theory suggests that conventional chemotherapies kill differentiated or differentiating cells, which form the bulk of the tumor but do not generate new cells. A population of CSCs, which gave rise to it, could remain untouched and cause relapse.*

Cancer stem cells were first identified by John Dick in acute myeloid leukemia in the late 1990s. Since the early 2000s they have been an intense cancer research focus. The term itself was coined in a highly cited paper in 2001 by biologists Tannishtha Reya, Sean J. Morrison, Michael F. Clarke, and Irving Weissman.

Metastasis

Metastasis is the major cause of tumor lethality. However, not every tumor cell can metastasize. This potential depends on factors that determine growth, angiogenesis, invasion, and other basic processes.

Treatment

CSCs are inherently more resistant to chemotherapeutic agents. There are 5 main factors that contribute to this:

1. Their niche protects them from coming into contact with large concentrations of anti-cancer drugs.
2. They express various transmembrane proteins, such as MDR1 and BCRP, that pump drugs out of the cytoplasm.
3. They divide slowly, like adult stem cells tend to do, and are thus not killed by chemotherapeutic agents that target rapidly replicating cells via damaging DNA or inhibiting mitosis.
4. They upregulate DNA damage repair proteins.
5. They are characterized by an overactivation of anti-apoptotic signaling pathways.

After chemotherapy treatment, surviving CSCs are able to repopulate the tumor and cause a relapse. Additional treatment targeted at removing CSCs in addition to cancerous somatic cells must be used to prevent this.

Targeting

Selectively targeting CSCs may allow treatment of aggressive, non-resectable tumors, as well as prevent metastasis and relapse. The hypothesis suggests that upon CSC elimination, cancer could regress due to differentiation and/or cell death.[citation needed] The fraction of tumor cells that are CSCs and therefore need to be eliminated is unclear.

Pathways

The design of new drugs for targeting CSCs requires understanding the cellular mechanisms that regulate cell proliferation. The first advances in this area were made with hematopoietic stem cells (HSCs) and their transformed counterparts in leukemia, the disease for which the origin of CSCs is best understood. Stem cells of many organs share the same cellular pathways as leukemia-derived HSCs.

A normal stem cell may be transformed into a CSC through dysregulation of the proliferation and differentiation pathways controlling it or by inducing oncoprotein activity.

My MRI's:

The day I had surgery 8/13/2013

From: TA:172.21.20.21:1720,TEL:912148   Page: 12/18   Date: 5/28/2014 11:58:05 AM
5/28/2014 11:44 AM   FROM: Fax Texas Neurosurgery LL2   TO: 1-901-322-2962   PAGE: 012 OF 018

BAYLOR

197641

DEPARTMENT OF PATHOLOGY
1500 Gaston Avenue
Dallas, TX 75246
Tel. # (214) 820-2251

Patient:	MCCRAW, JAMES A	Pathology. No.:	BDS-13-11280
MRN:	10149171 - 61010106	Date Collected:	8/13/2013
Patient Type:	A	Date Accessioned:	8/14/2013
Account No.:	61010106	Location:	3H - H0301 -A
Date of Birth:	1/7/1959	Service:	NEU
Sex: M	Age: 54	Attending Physician:	Christopher B. Micheal

SURGICAL PATHOLOGY REPORT

Specimen(s):
1. Left Brain Tumor
2. Left Brain Tumor

Additional Physician(s):
N. Bruce Jenseven
Gerald Murphy MD

Pre-Op Diagnosis: Left brain tumor.
Post-Op Diagnosis: See physician's progress notes.
Clinical History: 54-year old man with left brain tumor

GROSS DESCRIPTION:
1. The specimen is received fresh labeled "Mccraw, left brain tumor" and consists of multiple fragments of tan-pink tissue measuring 2.5 x 0.7 x 0.5 cm in aggregate. A portion of the specimen is submitted for frozen section analysis as (1FSA) yielding the diagnosis "Intermediate grade glioma" per Drs. Snipes/Thomas. (1FSA) is resubmitted as (1A). The remainder of the specimen is submitted in (1B).

2. The specimen is received in formalin labeled "Mccraw, left brain tumor" and consists of multiple fragments of tan-pink tissue measuring 2.5 x 1.0 x 0.5 cm in aggregate. The specimen is entirely submitted in (2A-2B).

VP:kw

MICROSCOPIC DESCRIPTION:
Permanent sections of the specimen submitted as "left brain tumor" confirm the diagnosis of infiltrating glioma. In both specimens, the tumor is moderately cellular and composed of fibrillated cells with hyperchromatic moderately pleomorphic nuclei. There are rare mitotic figures and focal microvascular proliferation adjacent to a region of calcification. The microvascular proliferation is only present in specimen 2.

Immunoperoxidase studies are performed. All controls show appropriate reactivity. The tumor is immunoreactive for mutant IDH1 (R132H), and the majority of the tumor cells show strong immunoreactivity for p53. NeuN highlights the neuronal architecture in the background. The MIB-1 labeling index is relatively low at approximately 2-4%.

BRAIN/SPINAL CORD: Biopsy/Resection

History of Previous Tumor/Familial Syndrome: None known

Specimen Type/Procedure: Resection

Baylor University Medical Center   *Department of Pathology*   Page 1 of 2

Baylor University Medical Center *Department of Pathology*

Specimen Handling:
- [X] Squash/smear/touch preparation
- [X] Frozen section
- [X] Unfrozen for routine permanent paraffin sections

Specimen Size: Greatest dimension: 2.5 cm
Additional dimensions: 2.0 x 2.0 cm (estimated aggregate)

Laterality: Left

Tumor Site: Brain, cerebrum

Histologic Type and Grade: Glioblastoma

Histologic Grade: WHO Grade IV

Margins: Not applicable

Ancillary Studies: Immunohistochemistry see above

Additional Pathologic Findings: Calcification, focal low grade features.

COMMENT:
This case was reviewed by Dr. L. Winneberger and by Dr. C. Goodman (Baylor College of Medicine SB-13-0638). Both felt that the majority of the tumor was more compatible with a grade III, but that the focal microvascular proliferation necessitates the diagnosis of glioblastoma. The IDH1(R132H) mutation is associated with a more favorable prognosis in glioblastoma.

DIAGNOSIS:
Brain, left brain tumor, biopsy and excision (Parts 1 & 2):
    Glioblastoma (WHO Grade IV)
    Mutant IDH1(R132H) detected

Final Diagnosis by George J. Snipes MD, PhD
8/22/2013 5:03:21PM

The electronic signature indicates that the named Attending Pathologist has evaluated the specimen referred to in the signed section of the report and formulated the diagnosis therein.

Patient:	MCCRAW, JAMES A			Pathology No.	BUS-13-11280
MRN:	10149171 - 61010106	Account No.:	61010106	Attending MD:	Christopher B. Michael
Date of Birth:	1/7/1959	Age: 54	Sex: M		

Cerner Imaging Exam Report
Facility: **GERMANTOWN**

Patient Name: MCCRAW, JAMES A
MRN: 50054040
FIN: 82104871
Patient Type: Observation
Accession No: MR-13-0036687
Exam Date/Time: 11/25/2013 17:25
Ordering Physician: Jensen , Deborah , APN FNP
Resident:
Interpreting Physician: Somogyi , Christopher Todd, MD
Reason for Exam: CA

DOB/Age/Sex: 1/7/1959 57 Years Male
Location: 4XHG/ 04/ A0
Exam: MRI Brain & Stem W/WO Cont
Exam Status: Completed
Transcriptionist:
Report Status: Final
Transcribed Date/Time:

READ
EXAMINATION: MRI BRAIN & STEM W/WO CONT: 11/25/2013 12:23 PM, MR130036687

CLINICAL HISTORY: CA

COMPARISON: Outside examination performed 11/18/2013

FINDINGS: Multiple pulse sequences and multiple imaging planes were acquired in the evaluation of the brain before and after the intravenous administration of 20 mL Magnevist contrast.

Postoperative changes are noted on the left. Specifically, a frontal craniotomy defect is present. Trace blood products are noted within and around the operative cavity. There is no evidence to suggest recent infarction.

The craniocervical junction is unremarkable. The upper cervical spinal cord is normal in appearance. The ventricles are normal in size and symmetry. Vascular flow voids are unremarkable.

A peripherally enhancing mass\residual tumor is again noted within the left frontal lobe measuring 3.5 cm x 2.3 cm x 2.6 cm. Additionally, ill-defined enhancement is also noted within the supratemporal region, best visualized on series 10 image 12, series 11 image 14 and series 12 image 3. Moderate surrounding vasogenic edema persists. Since the prior examination there has been no significant interval change. There are no new enhancing intra-axial masses identified.

IMPRESSION: The peripherally enhancing mass\residual tumor within the left frontal lobe has not changed significantly in size. Ill-defined enhancement is also noted within the supratemporal region on the left also compatible with residual and/or recurrent tumor. Moderate vasogenic edema persists also without significant change.

This report was dictated at Workstation ID: PLA3136

Dictation Date / Time: 11/26/13 8:08 am

Dictating Radiologist : Somogyi , Christopher Todd, MD

MRI Brain & Stem W/WO Cont   MCCRAW, JAMES A - 50054040

Most recent MRI (Carson)

Result type:	MRI Brain & Stem W/WO Cont
Result date:	July 14, 2014 9:59 AM
Result status:	Auth (Verified)
Result title:	MRI Brain & Stem W/WO Cont
Performed by:	Somogyi, Christopher Todd, MD on July 14, 2014 10:43 AM
Verified by:	Somogyi, Christopher Todd, MD on July 14, 2014 10:40 AM
Encounter info:	23632770, UNIVERSITY, Outpatient, 7/14/2014 -

Reason For Exam
CA

READ
EXAMINATION: MRI BRAIN & STEM W/WO CONT: 7/14/2014 9:15 AM, MR140023384

CLINICAL HISTORY: Brain tumor, follow-up examination

COMPARISON: 05/20/2014

FINDINGS: Multiple pulse sequences and multiple imaging planes were acquired in the evaluation of the brain before and after the intravenous administration of gadolinium contrast. Postoperative changes are again demonstrated on the left. Blood products are noted within and around the operative cavity, without interval change.

There is no evidence of diffusion restriction to suggest recent infarction. There is no evidence of intraparenchymal hemorrhage. The craniocervical junction is unremarkable. The upper cervical spinal cord is normal in appearance. The ventricles are normal in size and symmetry. There are no intra-axial masses identified. Vascular flow voids are unremarkable.

After the intravenous administration of contrast, subtle peripheral enhancement persists, surrounding the operative cavity, without interval change. Moderate edema is again demonstrated surrounding the operative cavity, without change. The previously described small enhancing focus, inferior to the operative cavity is again demonstrated and has not changed significantly in size. There are no new enhancing intra-axial lesions identified.

IMPRESSION: Postoperative changes are again demonstrated on the left. This been no significant interval change in the appearance of the small enhancing focus inferior to the operative cavity. Continued follow-up is recommended to document stability.

This report was dictated at Workstation ID: PLA1144

Printed by: Thomas, Kimberly M
Printed on: 7/14/2014 2:23 PM

This report was dictated at Workstation ID: PLA3139

Dictation Date/Time: 01/19/14 2:31 pm

Dictating Radiologist : Taylor, Eddie Lee, MD
Signing Radiologist : Taylor, Eddie Lee, MD
Final Signed Date/Time: 01/19/14 2:28 pm

*************** Final Signature Line ***************

*** END OF REPORT ***

Cerner Imaging Exam Report
Facility: **UNIVERSITY**

Patient Name: MCCRAW, JAMES A
MRN: 50054040
FIN: 26323862
Patient Type: Outpatient
Accession No: MR-14-0043301
Exam Date/Time: 12/15/2014 10:39
Ordering Physician: Lawson, Ronald David, MD
Resident:
Interpreting Physician: Selvidge, Sidney D, MD
Reason for Exam: Other, Enter in Comments

DOB/Age/Sex: 1/7/1959 57 Years Male
Location: IRADDCM/ /
Exam: MRI Brain & Stem W/WO Cont
Exam Status: Completed
Transcriptionist:
Report Status: **Final**
Transcribed Date/Time:

ADDENDUM
CORRECTION:

There is a transcription error in the original report. Please see the corrected portion of the report below, with the correction in bold.

FINDINGS: Postoperative changes are present on the left. Focal encephalomalacia is present in the left frontal lobe with minimal adjacent enhancement within the operative bed, unchanged from the prior study. Surrounding FLAIR hyperintense edema/infiltration persists, unchanged. Wallerian degeneration of the left corticospinal tract is again noted.

There is no restricted diffusion to suggest recent ischemia. There is periventricular signal hyperintensity on FLAIR imaging. There is no midline shift. There is no evidence of recent hemorrhage. The visualized paranasal sinuses and mastoid air cells are clear.
This report was dictated at Workstation ID: PLA1146

Dictation Date / Time: 04/24/15 11:03 am

Dictating Radiologist : Selvidge, Sidney D, MD
Signing Radiologist : Selvidge, Sidney D, MD
Final Signed Date/Time: 04/24/15 11:00 am

****** Final Electronic Signature Line *******

READ
EXAMINATION: MRI BRAIN & STEM W/WO CONT, 12/15/2014 10:00 AM, MR140043301

CLINICAL INFORMATION: Glioblastoma.

COMPARISON: MRI brain 9/15/2014

TECHNIQUE: Multiplanar/multisequence imaging of the brain was performed prior to and after the intravenous administration of 20 cc Magnevist contrast media.

Page 1Continued...

Cerner Imaging Exam Report
Facility: UNIVERSITY

Patient Name: MCCRAW, JAMES A
MRN: 50054040
FIN: 29746145
Patient Type: Outpatient
Accession No: MR-15-0014191
Exam Date/Time: 4/24/2015 09:56
Ordering Physician: Lawson, Ronald David, MD
Resident:
Interpreting Physician: Selvidge, Sidney D, MD
Reason for Exam: Other, Enter in Comments

DOB/Age/Sex: 1/7/1959 57 Years Male
Location: IRADDCM/ /
Exam: MRI Brain & Stem W/WO Cont
Exam Status: Completed
Transcriptionist:
Report Status: Final
Transcribed Date/Time:

READ

EXAMINATION: MRI BRAIN & STEM W/WO CONT, 4/24/2015 9:30 AM, MR150014191

CLINICAL INFORMATION: Glioblastoma.

COMPARISON: MRI brain 12/15/2014

TECHNIQUE: Multiplanar/multisequence imaging of the brain was performed prior to and after the intravenous administration of 20 cc Magnevist contrast media.

FINDINGS: Postoperative changes are again noted on the left. Left frontal postoperative encephalomalacia is present. A minimal degree of marginal enhancement persists, unchanged. Adjacent FLAIR hyperintense edema infiltration persists and also appears essentially unchanged. There is stable Wallerian degeneration of the left cortical spinal tract.

There is no restricted diffusion to suggest acute ischemia. There is normal appearing anatomy at the craniocervical junction. FLAIR imaging also demonstrates benign chronic periventricular signal hyperintensity, unchanged. There is no midline shift. Normal void signal is present in the internal carotid and basilar arteries. There is no evidence of recent hemorrhage.

The visualized paranasal sinuses and mastoid air cells are clear

IMPRESSION: Stable exam.

This report was dictated at Workstation ID: PLA1146

Dictation Date / Time: 04/24/15 11:00 am

Dictating Radiologist : Selvidge, Sidney D, MD
Signing Radiologist : Selvidge, Sidney D, MD
Final Signed Date/Time: 04/24/15 10:57 am

****** Final Electronic Signature Line *******
*** END OF REPORT ***

Cerner Imaging Exam Report
Facility: UNIVERSITY

Patient Name: MCCRAW, JAMES A
MRN: 50054040
FIN: 33683366
Patient Type: Outpatient
Accession No: MR-15-0030099
Exam Date/Time: 8/25/2015 10:37
Ordering Physician: Lawson, Ronald David, MD
Resident:
Interpreting Physician: Buechner, David E., MD
Reason for Exam: Other, Enter in Comments

DOB/Age/Sex: 1/7/1959 57 Years Male
Location: 1RADDCM//
Exam: MRI Brain & Stem W/WO Cont
Exam Status: Completed
Transcriptionist:
Report Status: Final
Transcribed Date/Time:

READ

EXAMINATION: MRI BRAIN & STEM W/WO CONT: 8/25/2015 10:15 AM, MR150030099

CLINICAL HISTORY: CNS neoplasm.

Technical: Sagittal, axial, and coronal imaging was performed using multi echo precontrast technique. Additionally, postcontrast T1-weighted axial and coronal imaging was obtained.

20 cc of Magnevist was administered IV.

FINDINGS: There are postoperative changes from previous left frontal craniotomy and left frontal tumor resection. There is operative encephalomalacia as well as gliosis in the left frontal lobe.

Postcontrast images demonstrate very minimal subjacent enhancement just at the inferior margins primarily of the local left frontal operative resection site. This specific finding appears very similar to the previous examination of April 24, 2015. Given the stable/unchanged imaging findings this is likely reflective of postoperative/post therapeutic type change.

No worsening areas of intracranial enhancement to suggest definite residual tumor is identified.

No new intracranial enhancing metastatic lesions are identified.

There is chronic nodularity and degeneration of the left corticospinal tract.

There is minimal inferiorly age proportionate supratentorial white matter degenerative type change.

IMPRESSION:
1. Postoperative changes from previous left frontal craniotomy and left frontal tumor resection. There is some residual minimal parenchymal enhancement just primarily inferiorly posterior to the local left frontal operative resection margins, unchanged from the previous study (April 20, 2015). Given the stable imaging findings, again this is most likely on a simple postoperative/post therapeutic type change.
2. No evidence of definite recurrent tumor.

This report was dictated at Workstation ID: PLA1132

Dictation Date / Time: 08/25/15 12:37 pm

MRI Brain & Stem W/WO Cont   MCCRAW, JAMES A - 50054040

Result Type:	MRI Brain & Stem W/WO Cont
Result Date:	December 15, 2015 9:16 AM
Result Status:	Auth (Verified)
Result Title:	MRI Brain & Stem W/WO Cont
Performed By:	Buechner, David E, MD on December 15, 2015 11:59 AM
Verified By:	Buechner, David E, MD on December 15, 2015 11:56 AM
Encounter info:	40632260, UNIVERSITY, Outpatient; 12/15/2015 - 12/15/2015

197641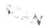

Reason For Exam
CA

READ
EXAMINATION: MRI BRAIN & STEM W/WO CONT: 12/15/2015 9:00 AM, MR150044426

CLINICAL HISTORY: CA , CNS neoplasm. Tumor.

Technical: Sagittal and axial imaging was performed using multi echo precontrast technique. Additionally, postcontrast T1 weighted axial and coronal imaging was obtained.

10 cc of Gadavist was administered IV.

FINDINGS: Comparison is made to the previous study of August 25, 2015.

There are postoperative changes from previous left frontal craniotomy and left frontal tumor resection. There is focal operative encephalomalacia and subjacent gliosis at the local left frontal operative resection site.

Postcontrast images do demonstrate some marginal enhancement particularly at the posterior and inferior operative margins. There has been some slight increase in amount of nodular enhancement at this location when compared to the previous study of August 25, 2015. The focal nodular enhancement now at the posterior inferior operative margins now measures approximately 1 cm in its superior to inferior extent and approximately 6 mm transversely. Slight worsening is best on postcontrast coronal imaging. With the slight worsening, findings would be suspect for a component of recurrent tumor. There has not been worsening in the vasogenic edema or other ancillary findings at this location.

No additional areas of abnormal parenchymal enhancement are identified.

There is abnormal elevated signal extending through the left corticospinal tract best depicted on posterior limb internal capsule and cortical spinal tract the level of the left mesencephalon representing Wallerian degeneration.

IMPRESSION:
1. Postoperative changes from previous left frontal craniotomy and tumor resection.
2. Slight worsening in nodular enhancement posterior inferior operative margins relative to previous studies. Findings would therefore be suspect for subtle component of recurrent tumor.

Printed by:	Fenton, Moon J, MD
Printed on:	12/23/2015 2:51 PM

WEST CANCER CENTER
7945 Wolf River Blvd.
Germantown, TN 38138
Telephone: 901-683-0055
Fax: 901-685-9718

Name: Mr JAMES A MCCRAW
DOB: 1/7/1959
Chart #: 197641
Physician: Christopher Boals
Date of Service: 2/17/2016 12:00 AM
Order No: 30954499
Ordering Physician: Moon J Fenton

Procedure: MRI of the brain with and without contrast

Reason for Study: Glioblastoma multiforme diagnosed in August 2013 status post surgical resection at an outside institution. Patient has been on maintenance Temodar. Most recent study at Methodist Hospital December 15, 2015 demonstrated suspected recurrent tumor. Followup.

Previous Examination: 12/15/2015 at Methodist Hospital

Findings: Axial T1, T2, FLAIR, and diffusion-weighted imaging with ADC map. The patient then received IV gadolinium (20 mL Omniscan) with post contrast T1-weighted imaging in all 3 planes. Postoperative changes in the left frontal lobe from remote tumor resection are stable, as is associated adjacent surrounding gliosis. There has been increase in size of the previously identified focus of nodular enhancement along the inferoposterior aspect of the surgical margin, now measuring 9.5 mm transverse by 8.9 cm craniocaudal by 5.1 cm AP, previously 6.3 x 8.5 x 5.2 mm.

There is no restricted diffusion to suggest an acute infarct. There is no hydrocephalus, extra-axial fluid collection, or intracranial hemorrhage. There is minimal right to left midline shift due to postoperative encephalomalacia. Intracranial flow voids are grossly unremarkable. Midline structures are unremarkable. Orbital contents are symmetric and unremarkable. There is mucosal thickening in the inferior left maxillary sinus. Remaining imaged paranasal sinuses and mastoid air cells are clear.

Impression:
1. Worsening recurrent disease along the inferoposterior margin of the left frontal resection site.
2. Left maxillary sinus disease.

THIS REPORT WAS INTERPRETED AT THE WEST CLINIC
Report Electronically Signed by: Christopher Boals

Semmes-Murphey Clinic
6325 Humphreys Blvd Memphis, TN 38120
(901) 522-7700 Fax:

March 14, 2016
Imaging Report

James A McCraw
Male DOB: 01/07/1959 PID: 240098   Ins: Medicare Tennessee

Home: (901) 585-0136

03/14/2016 - Imaging Report: MRI of the head before and after IV contrast. 20 cc of Omniscan
Provider: L Madison Michael
Location of Care: Semmes-Murphey Clinic
Status: UNSIGNED DOCUMENT

MRI of the head before and after IV contrast. 20 cc of Omniscan was
ORDER: 498873-2

PATIENT: McCraw, James
PATIENT ID: 240098
DATE OF BIRTH: 01/07/1959

EXAMINATION: MRI of the head before and after IV contrast. 20 cc of Omniscan was
injected intravenously.

Clinical: Glioblastoma, postop

There has been previous left frontal craniotomy with resection of intra-axial tumor.
Local encephalomalacia, gliosis, hemosiderin deposit and postoperative enhancement are
present at the site of tumor resection. Along the posterior margin of tumor resection
there is a 6 by 8mm nodular area of enhancement. No previous studies are currently
available for comparison of change but this appearance is very suspicious for recurrent
tumor. There is dilation of the left lateral ventricle adjacent to the site of tumor
resection and a component of Wallerian degeneration appears to involve the left
midbrain.

Overall ventricular size is normal and the ventricles are midline in location. There is
no evidence of recent infarction or recent hemorrhage. Normal flow voids are present in
the internal carotid arteries and basilar artery.

Impression postoperative changes on the left with probable recurrent tumor

Electronically Authenticated by RADIOLOGIST: Robert Laster, M.D.
REPORT:
03/14/2016_____

Semmes-Murphey Clinic
6325 Humphreys Blvd Memphis, TN 38120
(901) 522-7700 Fax:

May 24, 2016
Imaging Report

James A McCraw
Male DOB: 01/07/1959 PID: 240098 Ins: Medicare Tennessee

Home: (901) 585-0136

05/16/2016 - Imaging Report: MRI of the head before and after IV contrast. 20 cc of Omniscan
Provider: L Madison Michael
Location of Care: Semmes-Murphey Clinic

MRI of the head before and after IV contrast. 20 cc of Omniscan was
ORDER: 519726-1

PATIENT: McCraw, James
PATIENT ID: 240098
DATE OF BIRTH: 01/07/1959

EXAMINATION: MRI of the head before and after IV contrast. 20 cc of Omniscan was
injected intravenously.

Clinical: Glioblastoma, postop

Comparison: The study is compared to a previous MRI of March 14, 2016.

There has been previous left frontal craniotomy with resection of intra-axial tumor in
the left frontal lobe. There is a cystic cavity as well as gliosis, hemosiderin deposit
and postoperative enhancement at the site of tumor resection. The nodular enhancement
present on the previous exam has diminished compared to the previous study. The size of
the cystic cavity rim of enhancement is unchanged area. There is a small extra-axial
fluid collection on the left. This is stable. There is dilation of the left lateral
ventricle. The ventricles are midline in location. There is no evidence of recent
hemorrhage or recent infarction or new enhancing mass lesion.

Impression: Interval improvement.

Electronically Authenticated by RADIOLOGIST: Robert Laster, M.D.
REPORT: 05/16/2016

Electronically signed by L Madison Michael on 05/20/2016 at 4:32 PM

Semmes-Murphey Clinic
6325 Humphreys Blvd   Memphis, TN 38120
(901) 522-7700 Fax:

September 9, 2016
Page 1
Imaging Report

James A McCraw
Male DOB: 01/07/1959   PID: 240098   Ins: Medicare Tennessee   Home: (901) 585-0136

08/29/2016 - Imaging Report: MRI of the head before and after IV contrast. 20 cc of Omniscan
Provider: L Madison Michael
Location of Care: Semmes-Murphey Clinic

MRI of the head before and after IV contrast. 20 cc of Omniscan was
ORDER: 553894-2

PATIENT: McCraw, James
PATIENT ID: 240098
DATE OF BIRTH: 01/07/1959

EXAMINATION: MRI of the head before and after IV contrast. 20 cc of Omniscan
was
injected intravenously. Stealth protocol was included.

Clinical: Glioblastoma, postoperative status

COMPARISON: The study is compared to a previous MRI of May 16, 2016.

There has been previous left frontal craniotomy with resection of intra-axial
left
frontal lobe tumor. There is local gliosis, hemosiderin deposit,
encephalomalacia and
postoperative enhancement at the site of tumor removal. There is further
reduction in
the cystic cavity as well as the adjacent nodular enhancement compared to the
last exam
of May 2016. There is no suggestion of recurrent tumor growth since the
previous study.

There is supratentorial atrophy. There is dilation of the left lateral
ventricle
adjacent to the site of tumor resection. Overall ventricular size is normal
and the
ventricles are midline in location. Normal flow voids are present in the
internal
carotid arteries and basilar artery.

IMPRESSION: Interval improvement.

Electronically Authenticated by RADIOLOGIST: Robert Laster, M.D.
REPORT: 08/29/2016

Electronically signed by L Madison Michael on 08/29/2016 at 1:56 PM

Semmes-Murphey Clinic
6325 Humphreys Blvd Memphis, TN 38120
(901) 522-7700 Fax:

December 7, 2016
Imaging Report

James A McCraw
Male DOB: 01/07/1959 PID: 240098   Ins: Medicare Tennessee

11/28/2016 - Imaging Report: MRI of the head before and after IV contrast. 15 cc of Omniscan
Provider: L Madison Michael MD
Location of Care: Semmes-Murphey Clinic

MRI of the head before and after IV contrast. 15 cc of Omniscan was
ORDER: 384827-2

PATIENT: McCraw, James
PATIENT ID: 240098
DATE OF BIRTH: 01/07/1959

EXAMINATION: MRI of the head before and after IV contrast. 15 cc of Omniscan was
injected intravenously.

Clinical: Brain tumor, postop

COMPARISON: The study is compared to previous MRIs of August 29, 2016 and March 14, 2016.

There has been previous left frontal craniotomy with resection of intra-axial tumor in
the left frontal lobe. There is local encephalomalacia, gliosis, hemosiderin deposit and
postoperative enhancement at the site of tumor removal. Two nodular areas of enhancement
along the posterior margin of tumor resection have almost completely resolved compared
to the previous study of August 29, 2016. There is no new abnormal area of enhancement.
There is dilation of the adjacent left lateral ventricle which is unchanged. Additional
enhancement along the margin of tumor resection has diminished.

The remainder of the study continues normal with no evidence of infarction, recent
hemorrhage or new enhancing mass lesion. The ventricles are midline in location and
overall ventricular size is normal.

IMPRESSION: Interval improvement.

Electronically Authenticated by RADIOLOGIST: Robert Laster, M.D.
REPORT: 11/28/2016

Electronically signed by L Madison Michael MD on 11/30/2016 at 12:37 PM

PATIENT: McCraw, James
PATIENT ID: 240098
DATE OF BIRTH: 01/07/1959

EXAMINATION: Pre- and Postcontrast Brain MRI

HISTORY:
Follow-up glioblastoma treated by surgery, radiation therapy and chemotherapy

Technique:
Sagittal T1 W scans and axial T1 W, FSE T2 W, FLAIR T2 W, susceptibility weighted, and diffusion weighted scans of the brain with ADC map were performed on a 1.5 T system. Following IV Gadolinium contrast infusion (15 cc of Omniscan) sagittal, axial, and coronal T1-weighted scans of the brain were performed.

Reference exam:
None available

Findings:
Acute intracranial hemorrhage - negative
Acute infarction - negative
Intracranial mass or mass effect - negative

Postoperative changes laterally and inferiorly in the left frontal lobe are stable. On 8/29/2016 there was a small area of nodular enhancement along the posterior medial aspect of the operative cavity. The enhancing area was smaller on 11/28/2016 and is stable today. A thin rim of enhancement along the remaining margins of the surgical cavity is consistent with postoperative change and is stable, also. T2 hyperintensity extending into subcortical white matter adjacent to the operative cavity as well as into the corona radiata and centrum semiovale is stable. There is no mass effect in this area. Compensatory enlargement of the left lateral ventricle is stable. There are no findings to indicate macroscopic recurrent tumor.

Wallerian degeneration extending along the cortical spinal tract into the cerebral peduncle is stable. No new signal intensity abnormalities are apparent in the brain. There are no new areas of intracranial contrast enhancement. Signal voids are visible in the intracranial internal carotid arteries bilaterally and in the basilar artery implying patency.

Opinion
Stable postoperative changes laterally and inferiorly in the left frontal lobe with no findings indicative of macroscopic recurrent tumor; no new intracranial abnormalities

This report was electronically signed by Dr. Craig Nauert 3/7/2017 1:39 PM
Workstation: MSIT-SMMQPS

Electronically Authenticated by RADIOLOGIST: Timothy Nauert, M.D.
REPORT: 03/07/2017

Summary: Image Report: MRI with and without contrast
Patient Name: James A McCraw
DOB:1/7/1959
Sex: M
MRN:EMR

Summary: MRI with and without contrast
MRI with and without contrast
ORDER: 708326-1

PATIENT: McCraw, James
PATIENT ID: 240098
DATE OF BIRTH: 01/07/1959

EXAMINATION: MRI with and without contrast

History:
58-year-old male with left frontal GBM, left frontal craniotomy and subtotal resection
August 20, 2013. Postoperative radiation therapy and concomitant chemotherapy.

Reference
Enhanced brain MRI 7/25/2017 and 6/12/2017

Technique
Routine enhanced brain MRI including sagittal and axial T1-weighted, axial FLAIR and
T2-weighted, axial susceptibility weighted, axial diffusion weighted, and enhanced sagittal, axial, and coronal T1-weighted imaging. In addition, enhanced axial T1 3-D
volume acquisition is obtained.

Findings
Left frontal postoperative changes of tumor resection again observed, grossly stable.
The resection cavity is unchanged in appearance. Surrounding T2/FLAIR hyperintensity is

also grossly unchanged. Previously observed 2 nodular foci of enhancement along the
lateral margin of the left lateral ventricle are improved/smaller from prior study. The
more posterior lesion shows the greatest improvement, nearly resolved. There is no new
abnormal enhancement observed. No developing mass effect is apparent. There is no new
signal abnormality within the brain or brainstem.

There is no hydrocephalus, mass effect, or extra-axial fluid collection. The orbits and
skull base are grossly unremarkable.

Impression
Improved nodular enhancing foci along the lateral margin of the left lateral ventricle.
No additional interval change.

This report was electronically signed by Dr. Scott Didier 11/6/2017 11:27 AM
Workstation: MSIT-SMMQPS

Electronically Authenticated by RADIOLOGIST: Scott Didier, M.D.
REPORT: 11/06/2017

Signed by L Madison Michael MD on 11/6/2017 12:08:10 PM

--- Summary: Imag Rpt: MRI with and without contrast
Patient Name: James A McCraw
DOB:1/7/1959
Sex: M
MRN:EMR

Summary: MRI with and without contrast

MRI with and without contrast
ORDER: 708326-1

PATIENT: McCraw, James
PATIENT ID: 240098
DATE OF BIRTH: 01/07/1959

EXAMINATION: MRI with and without contrast

History:
58-year-old male with left frontal GBM, left frontal craniotomy and subtotal resection
August 20, 2013. Postoperative radiation therapy and concomitant chemotherapy.

Reference
Enhanced brain MRI 7/25/2017 and 6/12/2017

Technique
Routine enhanced brain MRI including sagittal and axial T1-weighted, axial FLAIR and
T2-weighted, axial susceptibility weighted, axial diffusion weighted, and enhanced sagittal, axial, and coronal T1-weighted imaging. In addition, enhanced axial T1 3-D
volume acquisition is obtained.

Findings
Left frontal postoperative changes of tumor resection again observed, grossly stable.
The resection cavity is unchanged in appearance. Surrounding T2/FLAIR hyperintensity is
also grossly unchanged. Previously observed 2 nodular foci of enhancement along the
lateral margin of the left lateral ventricle are improved/smaller from prior study. The
more posterior lesion shows the greatest improvement, nearly resolved. There is no new
abnormal enhancement observed. No developing mass effect is apparent. There is no new
signal abnormality within the brain or brainstem.

There is no hydrocephalus, mass effect, or extra-axial fluid collection. The orbits and
skull base are grossly unremarkable.

Impression
Improved nodular enhancing foci along the lateral margin of the left lateral ventricle.
No additional interval change.

PRE AND POSTCONTRAST BRAIN MRI
ORDER: 850767-2

PATIENT: McCraw, James
PATIENT ID: 240098
DATE OF BIRTH: 01/07/1959

EXAMINATION: PRE AND POSTCONTRAST BRAIN MRI

HISTORY:
Follow-up status post resection left frontal glioblastoma with postoperative radiation therapy and chemotherapy

TECHNIQUE:
Sagittal T1 W scans and axial T1 W, FSE T2 W, FLAIR T2 W, susceptibility weighted, and diffusion weighted scans of the brain with ADC map were performed on a 1.5 T system. Following IV Gadolinium contrast infusion (17 cc of ProHance) sagittal, axial, and coronal T1-weighted scans of the brain were performed.

Following the standard diagnostic MRI, 1 mm 3-D axial T1 W scans were performed through the entire brain using Stealth protocol.

REFERENCE EXAM:
Pre and postcontrast brain MRI on 5/7/2018

FINDINGS:
Acute intracranial hemorrhage - negative
Acute infarction - negative
Intracranial mass or mass effect - negative
Extra-axial blood or fluid collection - negative

Stable postoperative changes laterally and inferiorly in the left frontal lobe with surrounding white matter T2 hyperintensity consistent with gliosis; stable ex vacuo expansion of the left lateral ventricle and third ventricle; no left hemispheric mass effect; stable 3 mm right to left subfalcine herniation due to volume loss in the left hemisphere

Stable chronic lacunar insult extending from the lateral aspect of the left thalamus into the corona radiata and area of suspected postoperative gliosis

Stable minimal enhancement in medial and lateral walls of the surgical bed, likely postoperative change

Signal voids are visible in the intracranial internal carotid arteries bilaterally and in the basilar artery implying patency.

The paranasal sinuses, orbits, and mastoid areas are unremarkable bilaterally on these routine scans of the brain.

Semmes-Murphey Clinic
6325 Humphreys Blvd Memphis, TN 38120
(901) 522-7700 Fax:

November 5, 2018
Imaging Report

James McCraw
Male DOB: 01/07/1959 PID: 240098   Ins: Medicare Tennessee

Home: (214) 534-4372

11/05/2018 - Imaging Report: PRE AND POSTCONTRAST BRAIN MRI
Provider: L Madison Michael MD
Location of Care: Semmes-Murphey Clinic

PRE AND POSTCONTRAST BRAIN MRI
ORDER: 850497-1

PATIENT: McCraw, James
PATIENT ID: 240098
DATE OF BIRTH: 01/07/1959

EXAMINATION: PRE AND POSTCONTRAST BRAIN MRI

HISTORY:
Follow-up status post resection left frontal glioblastoma with postoperative radiation therapy and chemotherapy

TECHNIQUE:
Sagittal T1 W scans and axial T1 W, FSE T2 W, FLAIR T2 W, susceptibility weighted, and diffusion weighted scans of the brain with ADC map were performed on a 1.5 T system. Following IV Gadolinium contrast infusion (17 cc of ProHance) sagittal, axial, and coronal T1-weighted scans of the brain were performed.

Following the standard diagnostic MRI, 1 mm 3-D axial T1 W scans were performed through the entire brain using Stealth protocol.

REFERENCE EXAM:
Pre and postcontrast brain MRI on 2/7/2018

FINDINGS:
Acute intracranial hemorrhage - negative
Acute infarction - negative
Intracranial mass or mass effect - negative
Extra-axial blood or fluid collection - negative

Stable postoperative changes laterally and inferiorly in the left frontal lobe with surrounding white matter T2 hyperintensity consistent with gliosis; stable ex vacuo expansion of the left lateral ventricle and third ventricle; no left hemispheric mass effect; stable 3 mm right to left subfalcine herniation due to volume loss in the left hemisphere

Stable chronic lacunar insult extending from the lateral aspect of the left thalamus into the corona radiata and area of suspected postoperative gliosis

Stable minimal enhancement in medial and lateral walls of the surgical bed, likely postoperative change

Signal voids are visible in the intracranial internal carotid arteries bilaterally and in the basilar artery implying patency.

The paranasal sinuses, orbits, and mastoid areas are unremarkable bilaterally on these routine scans of the brain.

OPINION:
1. Stable left frontal lobe postoperative changes and gliosis in surrounding white matter; no MR evidence of macroscopic tumor recurrence
2. Stable chronic lacunar lesion extending from the lateral aspect of the left thalamus into the corona radiata and area of suspected gliosis
3. No new intracranial abnormalities

Semmes-Murphey Clinic
6325 Humphreys Blvd Memphis, TN 38120
(901) 522-7700 Fax:

James McCraw
Male DOB: 01/07/1959 PID: 240098   Ins: Medicare Tennessee

05/01/2019 - Imaging Report: PRE AND POSTCONTRAST BRAIN MRI
Provider: L Madison Michael MD
Location of Care: Semmes-Murphey Clinic
Status: UNSIGNED DOCUMENT

PRE AND POSTCONTRAST BRAIN MRI
ORDER: 919414-1

PATIENT: McCraw, James
PATIENT ID: 240098
DATE OF BIRTH: 01/07/1959

EXAMINATION: PRE AND POSTCONTRAST BRAIN MRI

HISTORY:
Glioma

TECHNIQUE:
Sagittal T1 W scans and axial T1 W, FSE T2 W, FLAIR T2 W, susceptibility weighted, and diffusion weighted scans of the brain with ADC map were performed on a 1.5 T system. Following IV Gadolinium contrast infusion (15 cc of Dotarem) sagittal, axial, and coronal T1-weighted scans of the brain were performed.

REFERENCE EXAM:
Pre and postcontrast brain MRI on 11/5/2018

FINDINGS:
Acute intracranial hemorrhage - negative
Acute infarction - negative
Intracranial mass or mass effect - negative
Extra-axial blood or fluid collection - negative

There are stable postoperative changes laterally and inferiorly in the left frontal lobe where there is encephalomalacia and confluent T2 hyperintense signal in adjacent white matter consistent with gliosis. Ex vacuo enlargement of the left lateral ventricle is stable. FLAIR T2 W hyperintense signal extending into the posterior limb of the left internal capsule is stable. No new signal intensity abnormalities are apparent in the brain. The remainder of the ventricular system is within normal limits.

Postcontrast coronal T1 W scans show smooth, sharply defined linear enhancement around the margins of the surgical cavity consistent with postoperative change with no nodular enhancement or change in the appearance from the prior study. No abnormal intracranial contrast enhancement is apparent.

Signal voids are visible in the intracranial internal carotid arteries bilaterally and in the basilar artery implying patency.

The paranasal sinuses, orbits, and mastoid areas are unremarkable bilaterally on these routine scans of the brain.

Semmes-Murphey Clinic
6325 Humphreys Blvd Memphis, TN 38120
(901) 522-7700 Fax:

July 8, 2020
Imaging Report

James A McCraw
Male DOB: 01/07/1959 PID: 240098   Ins: Humana Medicare Advantage

04/01/2020 - Imaging Report: Brain MRI with and without contrast
Provider: L Madison Michael MD
Location of Care: Semmes-Murphey Clinic

Brain MRI with and without contrast
ORDER: 1053663-1

PATIENT: McCraw, James
PATIENT ID: 240098
DATE OF BIRTH: 01/07/1959

EXAMINATION: Brain MRI with and without contrast

History:
61-year-old male for follow-up of left frontal GBM. Previous subtotal resection and postoperative radiation therapy and concomitant chemotherapy.

Reference
Brain MRI 5/1/2019 and 11/5/2018

Technique
Routine pre and postcontrast brain MRI including sagittal and axial T1-weighted, axial FLAIR and T2-weighted, axial susceptibility weighted, axial diffusion weighted, and enhanced sagittal, axial, and coronal T1-weighted imaging.

Findings
Postoperative changes of left frontal tumor resection are again observed. The resection cavity is grossly unchanged in overall size and shape from prior 2 exams. Surrounding T2/FLAIR hyperintensity in the left frontal lobe white matter is also very similar to prior studies. The T2/FLAIR hyperintensity is minimally increased within the left frontal deep white matter with a new small focus of T2/FLAIR hyperintensity slightly more anteriorly in the anteromedial aspect of the left frontal lobe. There is no new or worsening mass effect. There is no masslike enhancement appreciated. Minimal curvilinear postoperative enhancement is grossly stable. There remains ex vacuo dilatation of the left lateral ventricle similar to prior exams.

Signal intensities in the remainder of the brain and brainstem are unchanged. There is no midline shift or extra-axial fluid collection. There is no diffusion abnormality. Intracranial internal carotid arteries and basilar artery demonstrate signal void implying gross patency. The orbits and base are grossly unremarkable.

Impression
Postoperative changes of left frontal lobe tumor resection largely unchanged. Surrounding T2/FLAIR hyperintensity is largely stable with only minimal increase anteriorly in the left frontal lobe deep white matter with a new very small focus of T2 hyperintensity observed, nonspecific. No masslike enhancement and no developing mass effect.

Semmes-Murphey Clinic
6325 Humphreys Blvd Memphis, TN 38120
(901) 522-7700 Fax:

James A McCraw
Male DOB: 01/07/1959   PID: 240098   Ins: Humana Medicare Advantage

within the operative cavity within the lateral aspect of the left frontal lobe. A smaller area of hemosiderin deposition is identified within the anterior medial aspect of the left frontal lobe. These were present on the previous study.

Flow voids are demonstrated within the basilar and internal carotid arteries implying patency.

Mucosal thickening is noted within the frontal, ethmoid, and maxillary sinuses.

IMPRESSION:
1. Previous left frontal craniotomy with resection of a left frontal lobe mass lesion with stable postoperative changes/contrast enhancement within the operative cavity when compared to previous studies dating back through 11/6/2017.

This report was electronically signed by Dr. David Morris 10/21/2020 2:43 PM
Workstation: MSIT-SMMQPS

Electronically Authenticated by RADIOLOGIST: Stephen Morris, M.D.
REPORT:
10/21/2020

Made in the USA
Columbia, SC
21 December 2021